NURSE STAFFING

A Practical Guide

reprinted from
**Nursing
Administration
Quarterly**

Barbara J. Brown
Editor

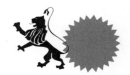

AN ASPEN PUBLICATION®
Aspen Systems Corporation
Germantown, Maryland
London, England
1980

Library of Congress Cataloging in Publication Data

Main entry under title:

Staffing.

"Reprinted from Nursing administration quarterly."
1. Nursing service administration—Addresses,
essays, lectures. 2. Health facilities—Personnel
management—Addresses, essays, lectures. I. Brown,
Barbara Jean, 1950- II. Nursing administration
quarterly. [DNLM: 1. Personnel administration,
Hospital—Collected works. 2. Personnel management—
Collected works. 3. Nursing, Supervisory—Collected
works. WY105 S778]
RT89.S65   610.73'068'3   80-12353
ISBN 0-89443-291-5

Library of Congress Catalog Card Number: 80-12353
ISBN: 0-89443-291-5

Printed in the United States of America

1 2 3 4 5

Contents

NURSE STAFFING

From the editor...

Staffing is the most written about, discussed, frustrated-over, agonizing situation, crucial problem, 24-hour dilemma confronting nursing service administrators today. Historically, it has been continuously dialogued as the most significant factor in creating the strong collective bargaining and economic security movement in nursing.

Staffing, the very complex multiple function responsibility of every nurse administrator, was chosen as a priority topic for concentration in this first year of NAQ's publication. Due to the nature of this complexity, we feel only a double-issue treatment of staffing could hope to cover the subject adequately.

Broadly defined, staffing is the complete personnel function of creating the staff and maintaining favorable conditions in which the staff works at optimum. It includes selection, orientation, training and development of nursing service personnel relevant to the delivery of quality patient care.

Staffing is the number one priority in creating a climate conducive to the professional practice of nursing. A nurse administrator can have nursing ideals intending to create a comprehensive delivery of nursing service as is evidenced in the primary nursing models.

However, if in reality there are insufficient numbers of RNs to provide comprehensive nursing care, it is illogical to think that comprehensive delivery of nursing service can occur. Several steps must first transpire before staff may be successfully expanded and comprehensive nursing service delivered. Nursing administrators must create a climate and environment conducive to the professional practice of nursing. The environmental element that causes the greatest concern is adequate funding for the hiring of numbers of nurses to allow for the professional practice of nursing to take place.

But what does one do then with the environment to create the proper climate? Climate is defined in three elements:

1. *Optimum freedom:* The freedom of individual nurses to fully implement the nursing process on every patient that they are assigned to.
2. *Energy release:* Leadership that enables individuals to maximize their potential in giving direction to decision making regarding the clinical practice of nursing.
3. *Statesmanship:* The key that creates the linkage to other units within the system that facilitates the professional practice of nursing.

Creating a suitable climate of operation is key to whether or not nursing personnel can be recruited and attracted to a setting and then indeed will be retained and maintained in that setting. It requires that all members of the group want and strive to achieve the objectives willingly and in keeping with the administrative philosophy for the delivery of nursing service.

To accomplish this, one must be cognizant of the human element in all decision making, and strive toward a participatory management system, enabling all staff nurses to give control to the staffing and the budgetary functions that relate to meeting their needs as well as the individual patient's needs.

This then means that we must find out what the individual employees' needs are and attempt to satisfy them so that the individuals can set their goals and feel comfortable about their accomplishments.

In staffing, we must also be concerned with the mutual interests of the total group, that is, the nursing staff on a particular unit. No individual works in isolation. Each person's goals are related to those of the group in which they work. Group satisfaction and acceptance is key to the staffing methodology that one uses. Each person depends upon the other when one is striving for unity of goal, plan and action.

There are a variety of staffing methodologies by which to achieve these principles. Each of these methodologies are interrelated and no one alone affords a total answer to the way in which staffing is or should be done. Methodologies discussed in Staffing: Parts I and II include:

- *Descriptive:* subjective judgment of values of variables and usually includes such things as census data, financial resources, comparative statistics, etc.
- *Industrial engineering:* assumptions made that nursing is a composite of tasks or activities and includes work distribution, work load factors as well as time and motion studies.
- *Management engineering:* nursing care provided represents quality desired. Patient classification is valid and nursing service demands should be distributed. Standard time of procedures is also valid and reliable. This forces us into a systems analysis looking at staffing and defining the various components such as personnel data and statistics, age of patient, cost figures, personnel skill levels, supportive services, numbers of patients, categories of patients and other variables.
- *Operations research:* studies and reports from industry utilizing mathematical allocation and situation models afford another

methodology relating to classes of patients, task complexes and cost values.

The movement toward an all-professional staff across the country forces nurse administrators to look at priorities in attempting such moves. Nursing process must be mandated to require that the direct care giver be a nurse, not a nursing assistant. With this mandate, there has to be a concentration on increasing the ratio of RNs to patients and diminishing nursing assistants' roles as direct care givers.

People who cannot perform according to the clinical expectations of excellence must improve their performance or be counselled to seek other areas of employment. By freezing positions for all personnel within nursing other than RNs when sufficient numbers of RNs have been recruited, ancillary positions should decrease in a normal way by attrition. In other words, it usually is not necessary to let valuable employees go but rather create a climate in which they may grow professionally. In some instances, nursing assistants and LPNs can be counselled into continuing education programs toward becoming an RN. Ideally, educational money should be available to assist these individuals in furthering their career goals. Such monies could have obligations to remain in the setting to contribute to patient care for a time period, thereby making it financially achievable.

Educational programs are key to creating a professional staff prepared to implement the full model of professional nursing. Therefore, comprehensive inservice programs are essential to the maintenance of staff. One such program is the recently developed nurse internship program. This certainly provides a mechanism to attract and stabilize new graduates to assist them in that transition from student to practicing professional nurse.

Recruitment mechanisms are key toward the selection of staff. Recruitment programs must be dynamic, creative, innovative, communicate the unique and distinctive role of nursing within an individual setting and should project a conceptual image to the public of what nursing is really all about.

Selection of staff should involve the effort of many people: personnel department and nurse recruitment working hand-in-hand with the nursing administrator having a final determination of who should join a staff that is committed to nursing excellence.

I frequently ask new graduates their philosophy of nursing: What do they want to accomplish with their patients? What are their goals for themselves as professionals? And will they really fit into the professional practice of nursing as we define it within our setting? With the best developed selection procedures, each of us occasionally selects a nurse that does not "fit in." It is our responsibility then to offer multiple alternatives to train, develop and counsel such individuals.

Barbara J. Brown, R.N., Ed.D.

Nursing Administration Quarterly
Editorial Board

Authors:

Luther P. Christman, Ph.D., R.N.
Vice President for Nursing Affairs
Rush-Presbyterian-St. Luke's Medical Center
Dean of the College of Nursing
Rush University
Chicago, Illinois

Jane N. Fairbanks, R.N., M.S.
Senior Instructor
University of Colorado School of Nursing
Assistant Director of Nursing
University of Colorado Medical Center Hospital
Denver, Colorado

Ruth Barney Fine, R.N., M.N., F.A.A.N.
Associate Professor
Community Health Services
School of Nursing
University of Washington
Seattle, Washington

Louis E. Freund, Ph.D.
Vice President
Medicus Systems Corporation
Chicago, Illinois

Alan L. Frohman, Ph.D.
Organization Consultant
Arlington, Massachusetts

Ethel Hill, R.N.
Assistant Vice President
Nursing Service
Bayfront Medical Center
St. Petersburg, Florida

Kaye Lillesand, B.S.N.
Director of Nursing Service
St. Nicholas Hospital
Sheboygan, Wisconsin

Laura L. Mathews, B.S.N.
Director of Nursing Service
Steven Bryant Nursing Home
Milwaukee, Wisconsin

Ronald B. Norby, R.N., M.N.
Director, Nursing Services
Medicus Systems Corporation
Chicago, Illinois

Joan O'Leary, R.N., Ed.D.
Vice President
Nursing Service
Bayfront Medical Center
St. Petersburg, Florida

Carol A. Smith, R.N., B.S.
Assistant Director of Nursing for
  Inpatient Services
The Children's Memorial Hospital
Chicago, Illinois

Eunice Lawrenz Smith, R.N., B.S.N.E.
Associate Consultant
Herman Smith Associates
Hospital Consultants
Hinsdale, Illinois

Gloria Swanberg, R.N., M.N.A.
Principal Consultant
Herman Smith Associates
Hospital Consultants
Hinsdale, Illinois

A Model for Nurse Staffing and Organizational Analysis

Ronald B. Norby, R.N., M.N.
Director
Nursing Services

Louis E. Freund, Ph.D.
Vice President
Medicus Systems Corporation
Chicago, Illinois

THERE ARE FEW universals in this world, but in talking with nurses throughout the United States, we are beginning to believe that at least one exists—a concern and dilemma regarding nurse staffing. While there are multiple reasons for this concern, a major factor lies in the fact that staffing becomes a focal point for multiple issues affecting nursing and the health care profession as a whole. As an example, two conflicting pressures are having a tremendous influence upon nurse staffing: 1) escalating costs for care delivery coupled with continual pressure for control, and 2) society's demands for more and better health services. Most of those involved in health care management feel this can only be achieved through efficient utilization of facilities and personnel. Consequently, the focus quickly becomes one of personnel management, and staffing falls at the head of the list where personnel are concerned. Since nursing personnel typically comprise over 50 percent of all hospital personnel, the onus falls upon the nursing department to efficiently manage this resource.

HIGHLY COMPLEX ISSUES

Nurse staffing is far from an easy concept to consider, for there are highly complex issues at hand and there has not been a great deal of innovation in the tools and approaches designed to provide assistance. Perhaps most important is the fact that the tools that have been applied have not always been realistic or acceptable to nursing. If there is any one lesson which can be learned from previous attempts to measure nursing workload for the purpose of decision making related to staffing and efficiently assigning personnel, it is, that in the final analysis, the case is very much in the hands of the nursing staff. In order for nurses to "buy into" and want to use any tools, models or methodologies, several conditions *must* be present.

First, the staff must agree that the approach addresses a real problem. Second, the approach must use measurements which are meaningful to nursing and, finally, solutions

If there is any one lesson which can be learned from previous attempts to measure nursing workload for the purpose of decision making related to staffing and efficiently assigning personnel, it is, that in the final analysis, the case is very much in the hands of the nursing staff.

generated by the approach must be presented in such a way that they are, indeed, realistic answers to the questions which require attention. The approach must also be flexible enough to deal with a myriad of special conditions related to problems and situations, such as competency and experience of individual staff members, special needs of individual patients, and so on.

RESOURCE MANAGEMENT PROBLEMS

There is absolutely no doubt that there are resource management problems in nursing at all levels and nurses need appropriate tools and approaches to assist in their decision making. Every day, head nurses and unit leaders make assessments of patient needs and staff capabilities and, using some model, create assignments in order to insure that appropriate care services are delivered. This process may be repeated several times during each shift as the situation changes. Also, each day, decisions are being made at an administrative level as to how many nursing personnel at each level of skill should be assigned to each patient care unit. Such allocation of personnel to units and the subsequent assignment each individual receives can vary widely in terms of workload. Thus, a huge process of resource management, occuring at several levels in the nursing hierarchy, happens each day in each institution. Throughout the nation, the vast majority of decision making in this process is based on the experience of those involved and their abilities to mentally juggle many complex factors to predict care workload and determine staffing requirements. This feat becomes monumental when one considers the fact that there are:

- **Non-routine, non-predictable occurrences:** Nursing units, as a rule, experience more than their share of unexpected events which drain staff time. Unexpected physicians' visits and orders, patients going "sour," interruptions from support departments and other nursing personnel, observation of previously unidentified patient needs, visitors and family, are among the many occurrences that the nursing staff must cope with each day. In addition, some "routine" things can quickly take on an air of uniqueness. Answering call lights, admitting and transferring patients, preparing patients for surgery or diagnostic tests all tend to confound traditional resource management techniques.

- **Variation of patients needs:** One necessary component for personnel resource allocation is an adequate description of the total requirements which must be accomplished. On a patient unit, patients' needs represent this component and categorization schemes exist today which effectively divide patients into groups according to their self-sufficiency. Although research has documented that nursing personnel

spend less time with self-sufficient patients than with total care patients, and that patient classification schemes are important to the staffing function, the implementation of these schemes has been widely avoided due to the time consuming process of obtaining the information required. In addition, the overall usefulness of end results is limited due to the unavailability of acceptable resource allocation models.

- **Overlapping skill levels:** There is no longer any doubt that tremendous overlap exists, in terms of capability for meeting certain patient needs, between RNs, LPNs and Aides. Resource allocation models have great difficulty in accepting and dealing with this fact, while practicing nurses know it as reality and must deal with it in decision making. Complicating this is the additional problem of role definition. It is still difficult to point to any single concept of the role of the RN, LPN and Aide which can be translated into concepts describing their capacity to accomplish patient care activities.

- **Varying individual competencies:** A great deal of the adequacy of a patient's care depends upon the individual competencies of the nursing staff; and nursing personnel categories are neither equal nor uniform. Differences are due to such factors as educational programs (there are several

4

different types of programs which prepare the RN), experience, motivation and other individual factors. For those addressing the resource allocation problem, this knowledge creates special difficulties. Personnel at each skill level should not be considered equal, yet most models require this assumption and leave sensitivity to differences up to the implementer. In practice, however, these individual differences in competency are extremely important variables and, hence, models which cannot accommodate them are largely ignored by nurses.

As previously mentioned, hospital costs are rising at a rapid rate and the availability of nursing personnel, at least in many areas of the country, is a major concern. Assurance that effective utilization of personnel is being achieved must be mandatory, and therefore, traditional methods of decision making must continually be challenged and improved upon where possible. What is needed are methodologies and techniques particularly responsive to nursing resource management which are acceptable to the nurses involved, actually obtain

---

What is needed are methodologies and techniques particularly responsive to nursing resource management which are acceptable to the nurses involved.

---

better solutions to problems than nurses can achieve without assistance and which have a foundation in theory that enables administration to more fully understand how this multifaceted resource is utilized at every level.

Perhaps of equal importance is that such methodologies not function in isolation but become an integral part of a larger analytical model. Too often, nurse staffing is considered as an end in itself. That is, efforts are directed solely at readjusting or otherwise providing individuals to cover workload. While important, this must be accomplished with consideration directed toward many other factors such as desired quality levels; goals related to allocation of responsibility for care delivery; the effect of staffing on morale, turnover and absenteeism; personnel cost; actual ability to meet workload, recruitment, etc.

Analyzing Relationships

The model presented in Figure 1 provides the ability to analyze relationships among multiple dimensions of the nursing department. It is solidly based on a methodology for nurse staffing which has on many occasions met the test of what we feel to be our most important critics—nurses themselves. This model enables those in leadership positions to document, analyze and problem-solve in the area of personnel utilization with full knowledge of how staffing decisions are affected by and impact other aspects of the department.

FIGURE 1. A MODEL FOR NURSE STAFFING AND ORGANIZATIONAL ANALYSIS

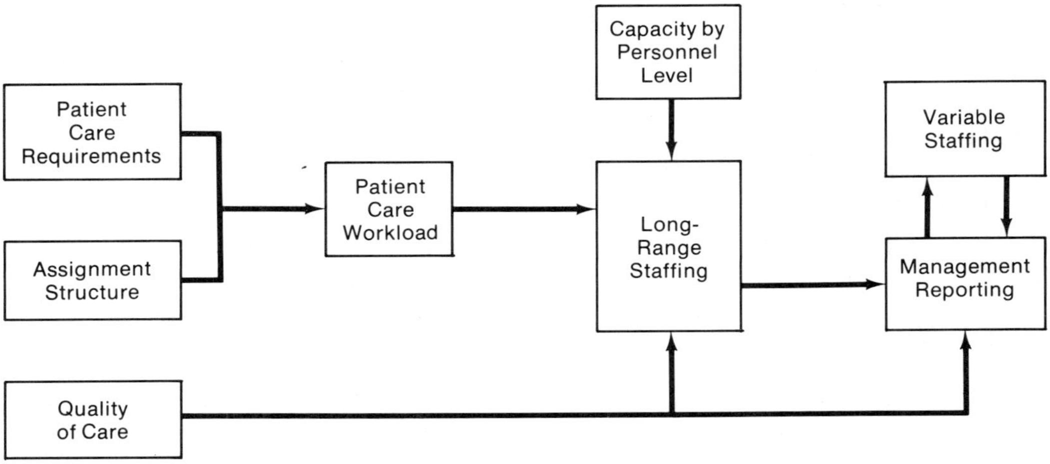

PATIENT CARE REQUIREMENTS

The questions of how many and what mix of nursing personnel are necessary to provide care services lead one into an extremely complex world of interactive variables. The temptation to simplify as much as possible (e.g., hours/patient day) or to standardize, ignoring substantial variance (e.g., RN hours/patient type), results in systems which are not too meaningful at an operational level.

The model which we propose reverses the questions. The key is individual patient care assignments which are constructed at the unit level by unit leadership personnel because such individual assignments reflect the impact of "staffing" decisions made by nursing administration. It is through the structure of assignments that unit leaders operationalize their

assessment of the balance between the number and types of staff available, individual competencies, self-sufficiency of patients, quality objectives, organizational approach, non-patient care responsibilities, interpersonal relationships and the myriad of other factors which are of importance.

Assignments vary from one day to another fairly widely for individual staff members. To confirm this, all you need to do is to informally ask a staff member "how's it going?" sometime toward the middle of the shift. Responses will generally range from "it's a really good day" to the extreme other end of the scale, "see me tomorrow, it's very bad today." Often, the same *number* of patients are present, but the workload associated with those patients varies dramatically due to the difficulty of the assignment. As suggested by this staffing model, the

6

assignment difficulty is dependent upon such factors as:

- The self-sufficiency (type) of patients in the assignment.
- The types of activities required by patients in the assignment.
- The number of patients of each category requiring each type of activity.

Assessing the Workload

Individuals' *perceptions* regarding assignment difficulty is, of course, also dependent on their experience, skill level, familiarity with the institution, support services available and so on. Hence, a method for realistically assessing workload in a quantifiable way must address these factors. Our experience has shown that this can effectively be done through a psychometric technique called constant-sum paired comparisons. Through the technique, each staff members' perceptions of the difficulty of each of the elements which might be used to structure their assignments can be addressed and a measurement of workload can be achieved.

Suppose, for example, that typical activity group structures (ways of communicating and assigning care) used on a nursing unit are:

- Medications (for a group of patients),
- Treatments (for a group of patients),
- Assessments (for each new admission), and,

- A.M. care (for a group of patients).

Staff members might have a combination of these activity groups assigned to them on any given day for a group of patients representing various levels of acuity. The model proposes that the more activity groups included in an assignment, and/or the more intensively ill the patients are for whom each activity group is required and/or the more patients for each included activity group, the more likely the assignment is going to be of high difficulty. Of course, lower difficulty assignments would be those with fewer activity groups and/or patients who are at a minimal dependency level, and/or very few patients at all.

So, with this approach to describing the assignments of personnel, which is developed, by the way, to be consistent with the practice and terminology actually used on each unit and shift, the question is not how many and what mix of staff should be provided, but what are the average numbers of each assignment element required by the patients and how should staffing progress in order that:

- Desired roles for each skill level (RN, LPN, Aide) are maintained in assignment structure.
- Total difficulty of assignments for each skill level does not vary from some specified optimum so as to negatively affect quality.

Answering these questions through implementation of the difficulty-based approach will generate meaningful staffing requirements which can be continuously managed.[1,2]

ASSIGNMENT STRUCTURE

Translating desired personnel roles (RN, LPN, Aide) into practice has been an extremely thorny problem for nursing managers. In this model, desired roles are reflected by the structure of personnel assignments for, in effect, the way care is assigned and delivered represents the agency's philosophy in action. To accomplish this, we clarify, for each skill level, the proportion of time each assignment structure (for patients at various levels of activity) *should* be assigned to RNs, LPNs and Aides. This is done by presenting a representative group of nurses with specific patient situations and asking them to indicate what personnel types should ideally be assigned to perform which of the assignment structures for each patient. Multiple patients are presented representing various acuity levels. The resulting set of proportions, developed for each shift, is referred to as a "Goals" matrix. It is a plan for the utilization of personnel which can be implemented at the unit level, since staffing recommendations are formulated around personnel required to fully implement the plan. In addition, by later collecting data as to the *actual* allocation of assignment elements to staff, the degree to which the goals matrix is being implemented can be monitored. It is possible then, to

7

It is possible to identify how and in what ways individual units and shifts are deviating from desired goals for care assignments to various personnel levels. Hence a type of vertical management control is established which has not previously been available in most nursing organizations.

identify how and in what ways individual units and shifts are deviating from desired goals for care assignments to various personnel levels. Hence a type of vertical management control is established which has not previously been available in most nursing organizations.

PATIENT CARE WORKLOAD

As previously mentioned, patient care workload for an individual staff member is related to the number and type of patients in an assignment and the activities (assignment components) provided. In order to quantifiably measure workload for staffing purposes, the model utilizes the psychometric technique, constant-sum paired comparisons. Greatly oversimplified, the technique proceeds as follows:

If, on a particular patient care unit, it is seen that there are four common assignment components (e.g., Medications, Treatments, A.M./P.M. Care, Assessments) and three levels of

8

patient acuity (as determined by classification), 12 assignment "elements" are constructed—one for each possible combination of patient type and assignment component (i.e., medications for self-care patients, treatments for intensive care patients, etc.). Each element is then paired with each other element and nurses are asked to judge the difference in difficulty between the two. These differences as perceived by nurses relate not only in the activities themselves, but also to the complexity of patient needs, priorities, consequences of error, skills and expertise required, time required per encounter and many other factors.

The premise is simple. The workload which results from being assigned to medications for self-care patients is different from that resulting from an assignment to medications for complete patients. How much less? The answer to that is measured for each personnel group on each unit and shift by asking the nurses to divide 100 points between the paired elements according to the difficulty of accomplishing one element as opposed to the other. A ratio scale of difficulty results with each element having a specific "value" for that unit, shift and personnel level.

During a one month data collection period, actual workload is calculated as nurses complete Patient Summary forms (each day and shift) to indicate what elements were required for patients (representing various levels of acuity) on the unit. Since there are

"values" for each element, it is only necessary to review desired roles to stipulate which personnel level *should* be expected to be allocated each required element. The sum of the difficulties for the elements allocated to RNs becomes the RN workload (in difficulty units), the sum of difficulties allocated to LPNs becomes the LPN workload, etc. Note that each personnel group has established its own scale through the questionnaire procedure.

QUALITY OF CARE

Most nursing departments have some method for assessing care quality. Measurement of quality is essential to the staffing function, for any decisions regarding staffing will have their ultimate effect on the quality of care services delivered. For this reason, we feel it is essential to assess quality from as many perspectives as possible, utilizing various tools and approaches to measure structure, process and outcome. From an operations analysis point of view, process measurement is essential in that it focuses on care delivery while in progress.

Most educators, practitioners and administrators will agree that the quality of nursing care is dependent on the number and types of patients on the unit as related to the numbers, types, and competency of available staff. As a result, the need for understanding of the interrelationships between these factors has long been a subject of discussion in the nursing literature. The majority of models suggest that high quality of nursing care should be the objective of every staffing decision.

Research has shown that lower quality care occurs as a result of both over and understaffing. Consequently, since the workload on a unit often varies dramatically from day to day, one rather naive management action to achieve high levels of quality is to add or delete personnel routinely to correct the workload/staffing relationship. In practice, some of this type of action occurs but, as many have found, as a steady diet, it begins to backfire. Continuity of care is jeopardized, the concept of "home unit" and "work groups" are routinely violated, and uncertainty on the part of staff about the situation can be high.

As a result, another balancing approach is frequently utilized first— that of changing the organization pattern to meet the situation. By organizing functionally, a high workload to staff ratio can be modified and presumably a higher quality of care can be delivered while some role concepts may be violated. By organizing a team mode, some role concepts are recovered, and quality can remain high. A primary nursing focus presumably permits the highest level of role concept and quality to be realized.

Of course, daily assessment and reorganization based on the workload/staffing situation is nearly impossible to bear. Hence, often one mode or the other is selected, and assignment content is varied to reflect the situation of the particular day. In practice, then, staffing decisions form only a part of the solution to a unit's problem of achieving maximum patient care quality. Quality measurement is essential to the model since it provides data of major impact to the management process.

CAPACITY BY PERSONNEL LEVEL

Workload can be converted to required FTEs for long-range staffing if one knows how much of the workload should ideally be assigned to each staff member. We refer to this as an individual's *capacity* for accepting workload. Obviously capacity must be related to some assumptions about over and underwork situations as they relate to quality of care objectives.

In the research from which the staffing methodology was developed, a tool was utilized to measure the quality of care services provided. This tool incorporates interviews with patients and staff as well as direct observations of the patient, the patient's records and the environment to assess the "process" of care delivery.[3,4] Assessment of care delivery was made repeatedly over the study period and was compared to the workload of the various staff members. The research documented the fact that when workload (as expressed in assignment difficulty) is low, the quality is likewise low. As

10

workload increases, care quality also increases up to a point at which further workload affects quality negatively. We find that nurses relate to this finding and generally agree that it is frequently validated in practice. The point at which quality and workload were optimally interrelated was identified as the capacity for each personnel type. *Capacity* then relates to that point at which maximum quality and workload are achieved. The research established average capacities per work shift of 2.75 for RNs, 2.50 for LPNs and 1.25 for Aides.

LONG-RANGE STAFFING

Long-range staffing recommendations (budgeted positions) formulated as data from the one-month study period are summarized and reallocated via the goals matrix; average workloads for each personnel level (specific to each unit and shift) are determined; and workloads are divided by appropriate personnel group capacities. The resulting FTEs are for the provision of *direct* patient care services.

Following this activity, discussions are held with nursing administration to determine desired administrative roles and hospital policies related to such areas as time off, holiday, vacation, etc. These factors are then added to FTE requirements for direct patient care. Since resulting FTEs are related to each unit, shift and personnel level, position control can be established at a very specific level which surpasses merely assigning a certain number of individuals to a particular unit.

VARIABLE STAFFING

In the development of a mechanism for determining day-to-day, shift-to-shift staffing requirements, the following are accomplished:

- Development of methods for daily calculation of unit workload.
- Initiating methods for identifying staffing needs and available resources.
- Constructing methods for daily data collection in relation to workload requirements and staffing adjustments.

During the initial phases of the staffing implementation, discussions are held with appropriate individuals to determine data processing capabilities and the availability of services. The approach to structuring the variable staffing, quality monitor-

---

The approach to structuring the variable staffing, quality monitoring and management reporting systems are developed to maximize existing resources, and data processing software is developed and installed as appropriate . . . multiple options are available for processing data.

---

ing and management reporting systems are then developed to maximize existing resources, and data processing software is developed and installed as appropriate. The staffing methodology itself is not dependent upon any particular level of computer support and multiple options are available for processing data.

TABLE 1

Sample Variable Staffing Output for Programmable Calculator

```
AUTO START

PROGRAM ?          Input Program Code
                                                    SHIFT  =              2.0
UNIT # ?           Input Unit Number                PERS. TYPE            1.0
        1.0                                                    10.0
VARIABLE STAFF                                                  0.2
SUMMARY                                                         3.8
CENSUS-MIX ?                                        PERS. TYPE            2.0    Night
CENSUS       30.0   Current Census                             5.9             Shift
TYPE 1       15.0                                              2.4
TYPE 2       11.0         # of pt.                  PERS. TYPE            3.0
TYPE 3        3.0        (each type)                           2.7
TYPE 4        1.0                                              2.2
ACUITY INDEX  1.7   Average Pt. Acuity              WORKLOAD  =          18.6


            Assessment   0.0                        SHIFT  =              3.0
Type I      A.M./P.M.   15.0                        PERS. TYPE            1.0
            Meds.       14.0                                   5.2
            Treatments   8.0                                   0.2
                                                               2.1
                         2.0                        PERS. TYPE            2.0    P.M.
Type II                 11.0                                   3.7             Shift
                        10.0                                   1.5
                         5.0    Summary of Required  PERS. TYPE           3.0
                         1.0    Assignment Groupings            1.0
Type III                 3.0                                   0.8
                         3.0                        WORKLOAD  =           9.8
                         3.0

                         0.0
Type IV                  1.0
                         1.0
                         1.0


        SHIFT  =        1.0     A.M. Shift
        PERS. TYPE      1.0     RNs
               12.6            RN Workload
                0.4            Administrative Factor
                5.0            Suggested RN Coverage
        PERS. TYPE      2.0     LPN
                4.5
                1.8
        PERS. TYPE      3.0     AIDE
                2.9
                2.3
        WORKLOAD  =    19.9     Total Unit Workload
```

When computer capabilities are not available, an efficient method for data processing is through the use of a programmable calculator. Cost for such a calculator is quite low and system control can easily be achieved within the nursing department. We have developed calculator programs for the data processing requirements of these systems which accept summary data or detailed data. In this manner, the staffing clerk can enter data directly from unit patient classification forms, and eliminate the need for summarizing data, which allows staffing to be calculated in a minimal amount of time. Programs have been developed for this calculator to compute staffing, allocate available staff, construct the management report and create quality scores. Table 1 shows a sample output from the calculator for variable staffing.

It is usually not necessary to collect workload data on all shifts in order to determine 24-hour staffing requirements. During the study period for which long-range staffing is calculated, data is collected in relation to the workload on all shifts. From this data, it is possible to utilize workload data from the day shift to predict workload on the evening, night and the following day shifts. Staffing requirements for these shifts are then calculated from the projected workload.

This predictive capability is tested during the implementation of the variable staffing component by comparing the prediction to actual workload. In all instances, we have achieved exceptionally high correlations. This fact in essence indicates the success of the predicting capability of the variable staffing system. In this manner, it is possible to free evening and night shift personnel from the added responsibility of completing data forms for the identification of daily workload on their shift.

Once staffing has been computed for each unit, this data is compared to the staff coverage which has been scheduled and discrepancies are noted. Some units will be shown to have adequate coverage while others will be shown as over or understaffed.

MANAGEMENT REPORTING

Significant is the fact that management reporting is last to be discussed in this article for it is the point at which elements of the model come together and analysis takes place. Each element of the model provides nursing management with specific data as input to the decision-making process. From identification of patient care requirements, information related to patient mix (by level of acuity) and assignment components is obtained.

Discussions around assignment structures reveal goals for care delivery and enable clarification of personnel roles. Workload data shows how care is actually distributed and how the workload is assigned among personnel levels. Capacity relates to optimal assignments for quality of care. Long-range and variable staffing show changing care delivery needs, changing workloads, and changing staff requests. Through quality care assessment, indications of levels of quality are identified.

The management report then, brings these and other data together for analysis and decision making. It goes without saying that the nursing department is totally interactive. Decisions in one area are certain to have their impact on other areas. Consequently, the goal of the management report is to provide a one-source document which creates a unit profile enabling comparisons of care quality, unit workload, census, staffing requirements, adjustments, actual staffing, illness/absence rates, overtime and other desired data.

As information is summarized on a monthly basis and compared to quality, a comprehensive picture of each unit is possible. Analysis of such data can show that original long-range staffing requirements for a given unit might have changed due to a general change in patient acuity levels or a change in average census. Such changes would be reflected in overall unit workload as well as staffing requirements reported on a regular basis. As reasons for the change are analyzed and compared to quality scores, decisions can be made concerning needed alterations in long-range staffing. Likewise, since data has been systematically collected, it is available to support necessary requests for budget deviations.

The model we have just discussed is rather comprehensive and goes far beyond traditional ways of looking at nurse staffing. The methodology for determining staffing needs has proven itself over and over as reliable, efficient, and acceptable to nurses and administrators. The fact that there are built in data collection and documentation protocols and that there is a mechanism for systematically organizing information (through the management report) allows for goal-directed decision making. This in itself is invaluable since decisions can be made with a maximum amount of data and solid facts as opposed to assumptions.

Perhaps most important to us is that the model has proven its value in nursing departments throughout the country. We have received many comments from those using the approach but there seems to be a central theme to the feedback; "for the first time, we've got a way of pulling all together in a way that makes sense to us as well as others."

REFERENCES

1. Freund, L. E. and Mauksch, I. G. "Optimal Nursing Assignments Based on Difficulty." USPH 1-R18-HSO1391 (Columbia: University of Missouri 1975).
2. Norby, R. B., Freund, L. E., and Wagner, B. "A Nurse Staffing System Based Upon Assignment Difficulty." (Chicago, Illinois: Medicus Systems Corporation 1977).
3. Jelinek, R. C., et al. A Methodology for Monitoring Quality of Nursing Care (DHEW: Pub. #HRA 74–75 Jan. 1974).
4. Haussman, R. K. D., et al. Monitoring Quality of Nursing Care (DHEW: Pub. #HRA 76–7 July 1976).

Adequate Staffing: It's More Than a Game of Numbers

Carol A. Smith, R.N., B.S.
Assistant Director of Nursing for
Inpatient Services
The Children's Memorial Hospital
Chicago, Illinois

STAFFING FOR QUALITY of patient care has long been a concern of nursing administrators, and certainly has been and is a concern for us at Children's Memorial Hospital. A little over a year ago, we found ourselves extremely short-staffed, utilizing large numbers of outside agency personnel to fill the gaps, asking our own staff to work many hours of overtime, and obviously providing less than optimal patient care. Motivated by our deep concerns regarding this situation, we felt a need to provide the quality of patient care we wanted and felt we were obligated to give.

As we began our undertakings, one thing was apparent: our traditional use of "nursing care hours," while readily available for projecting staffing requirements and the personnel budget, had given us less than optimal results in the past and we, therefore, did not want to use this method again if something better was available. We all had "gut feelings" as to what type of personnel we needed and what kind of mix (RN, LPN, Aide) we would like, but had no good concrete data to support and communicate our viewpoint to the administration or the Board of Directors.

We have reviewed staffing studies done at other children's hospitals in the United States and Canada.[1] Most of these institutions had utilized consulting firms to do time studies to help them identify their staffing needs. We had, in fact, done time studies of our own on two units to determine how much actual time it took to care for acute versus chronically ill children of all age groups.

Our experience had shown that this approach was extremely time consuming and after reviewing the experience of others, we felt the resulting data provided little meaningful information which could be utilized by our institution. Since we felt our situation was critical, time was a key factor and it became obvious that we could not find the answers ourselves without considerable time involvement effort. We therefore began looking for outside consultants to provide specific expertise and assistance.

FINDING ASSISTANCE

Wanting the very best assistance available, we reviewed several firms, looking in depth at their approach and services. This search led us to Medicus Systems Corporation who, fortunately, had their corporate offices in Chicago, and had worked with other hospitals in the Chicago area in nursing staffing and quality assurance. Due to this, it was possible for us to observe their work firsthand. After talking with and visiting several institutions where Medicus had provided services, we felt we would like to have them evaluate our situation and perhaps help us with our problem.

As a first step in developing a proposal, a multidisciplinary team of Medicus representatives visited the hospital and conducted interviews with individuals within our institution representing nursing, medicine, administration and staff development. These interviews were directed toward clear identification of our current situation as well as factors contributing to our problem. Following these interviews a proposal was submitted outlining Medicus' understanding of our problems and a suggested plan for action. Among objectives enumerated in the proposal were those leading to:

- Achievement of better management of staffing through workload monitoring.
- Reduction of the utilization of outside agency personnel.
- Improvement of the management skills of nursing administration.
- Introduction of quality of nursing care monitoring and obtaining baseline data.
- Development and implementation of nursing management information systems.

Having identified these needs and knowing what tools would be avail-

> *Since it is the philosophy of our department that as many people as possible should have a voice in change as it occurs, we proposed heavy participation by our staff in all aspects of the project.*

able, we established long- and short-term goals for the staffing project.

Since it is the philosophy of our department that as many people as possible should have a voice in change as it occurs, we proposed heavy participation by our staff in all aspects of the project. Although we would have a great deal of involvement by hospital and Medicus personnel, we felt that some one person within our nursing department was needed to act as coordinator for the project. This individual would actively participate and work as liason between those working within the institution and the consultants and would be a key individual for continuing the project at the end of outside support.

ESTABLISHING A STAFFING SYSTEM

The staffing system which was to be established at The Children's Memorial Hospital was aimed at providing a measurement of nursing workload as a basis for long-range and variable (daily) staffing. Workload determination is based upon the nursing activities performed in the actual delivery of nursing care to the patient. The amount of work associated with the performance of these activities is derived from the level of self-sufficiency of the patient and the nurse's perception of the difficulty of performing each activity.

To determine patient self-sufficiency, a classification tool needed to be developed specific to the care needs of children. Although Medicus had previously implemented patient classification systems in more than 50 hospitals throughout the United States and Canada, such a system had never been used in a total pediatric setting. Using a committee composed of four head and four staff nurses (representing medical, surgical, intensive care and infant care units) we looked at previously developed patient classification forms and realized that they wouldn't totally meet our needs.

After identifying usable portions from the forms, we struggled to construct our form by identifying common patient care needs based on the condition of the patient, the basic care each patient might require, and the therapeutic needs of a patient and/or his family. After several sessions and much discussion, we finally arrived at 34 "condition indicators" which would differentiate levels of patient acuity and would be applicable for any patient admitted to our hospital or any of our nine units.

We soon learned that agreeing on the list of indicators was the easiest part of the particular project. Coming to agreement on definitions for each indicator was much more difficult since we all had different opinions as

FIGURE 1. SAMPLE PATIENT SUMMARY FORM

18

Assignment Summary
- Specialing
- Monitor/Treatments
- Medications
- Routine Care

Unit: ___ Shift: ___ Date: ___ | Rm. No. | Patient's Name

Conditions
- Admission and Discharge
- Age: 0 to 8 Years
- Age: 8 Years to Adult
- Incontinent
- Disoriented/Retarded
- Blind or Deaf
- Isolation
- Partial Immobility
- Complete Immobility
- Severe Respiratory Distress
- Tracheostomy
- Surg.: Day of Surgery
- Surg.: 1 Day Post-Op

Basic Care
- Bed Rest
- Up With Assistance
- Bath With Assistance
- Bath Total
- Feeding: Oral With Assistance
- Feeding: Oral Total
- Feeding: Tube Total
- Feeding: Over 1/2 Hour Feeding
- Feeding: Frequency Q^{4n}

Therapeutic Needs
- I & O
- Specimen Collection
- Tube Care
- Suctioning Q^{4n}
- Wound or Skin Care
- Oxygen Therapy
- Vital Signs Q^{2}rr. or More
- Monitor up to Q^{15} Min.
- IV's
- Special Teaching Needs
- Special Emotional Needs
- Prepped for Procedure

to the meaning of specific terms. In order for the tool to be useful, we had to come to some consensus. The patient classification tool presented in Figure 1 is the result of that agreement.

Once we had established the format for the classification form, it was tested on the four units mentioned above. We quickly felt comfortable with the classification tool and expanded its use to all inpatient units. This expansion provided us with a clear example of the importance of including as many individuals as possible in changes as they occur. Implementation of the tool on all units meant a period of orientation for staff who were not originally involved in the tool's development. It was a little more difficult to "sell" the program to this group since they had less of a grasp of the reason behind the tool and tended to see only the fact that they were being asked to fill out additional forms. A great deal of orientation was needed for this group before they were able to "buy in" to the tool and recognize its worth. Once adequate data were collected to insure that the forms were being utilized correctly on all units, we were ready to move on to the next phases of the project—quality review and establishing workload measurement of each unit.

Determining Staffing Requirements

In the approach we utilized to determine staffing requirements, workload was not determined through the use of traditional time study tech-

In the approach we utilized to determine staffing requirements, workload was not determined through the use of traditional time study techniques . . . our approach was based on the concept of assignment "difficulty."

niques. While these approaches would add the number of elements to be accomplished on a particular unit, relate the element to patient type and multiply by the "standard time," our approach was based on the concept of assignment "difficulty."

As one looks at assignment elements (i.e., providing A.M. care for a group of critically ill patients, passing medications to a group of minimal care patients, etc.), it is apparent that some are more difficult to accomplish than others. Differences relate not only to what needs to be done to accomplish the element (i.e., provide A.M. care) but also difficulty relates to the level of acuity of the patient for whom an assignment element is performed.

Although time is certainly involved, other factors such as the skill and knowledge of the staff, organizational skills of the staff, their ability to problem solve, accessibility to supplies and equipment, usual methods of assignment, etc., contribute to the degree of difficulty of a task. Nurses are able to judge the difficulty of accomplishing one assignment element as compared to another.

In beginning to develop the method

20 to determine workload, therefore, staff were interviewed by members of the Medicus Staff to determine the structure of their usual assignment and "assignment elements" were developed (i.e., routine care for four patients). All combinations of elements were paired and staff were asked to complete questionnaires to determine their perceptions of the difficulty of accomplishing one element as compared to the other, if it were included in their assignment. For example, one pair was:

- Medications for two intensive care patients.
- Medications for five self-care patients.

Questionnaires were developed specific to each unit, shift, and personnel type (i.e., RN, LPN, Aide) and administered to a maximum number of personnel. Results of this questionnaire process then provided a numerical "value" for the difficulty of performing each assignment element, and values were specific to unit, shift and category of personnel.

QUALITY ASSURANCE

We felt that it was equally important when looking at the numbers of personnel required to relate this to quality of care. Quality assurance played an important role in the Medicus approach and it was imperative that we began assessing quality early as we needed to develop a baseline. Such a baseline would assist us in knowing what and if any

significant changes occurred in the quality of care as a result of changes in staffing and/or staff mix. Medicus proposed, and we agreed, that the most valid measure for comparing staff to the quality of nursing care is that which focuses on nursing activities performed in the actual delivery of nursing care to the individual patient: the process model of patient care. Medicus had previously developed a tool for measuring the quality of the care process and we chose to utilize this since it provided an assessment of direct care of the patient by the nurse and also the quality of support services in facilitating nursing care (i.e., unit management, dietary, etc.).

Again, we realized that to achieve acceptance, this must be done with available inhouse staff. The decision was made to train the already existing audit committee in conducting necessary observations based on the fact that they were (1) a group who was used to working together doing discharge outcome and auditing (chart review), and (2) the group was composed of head nurses and staff nurses representing several nursing units. The entire group of nine attended a three-day workshop on the system which for us not only involved learning the method of review but changing the wording of several of the questions to make them more oriented to a pediatric setting. During the month of March 1976, 178 reviews were done on all inpatient units for all three shifts—a commendable undertaking for a group of nine people who had other full-time commitments on their assigned units.

In March, we received the preliminary reports of our quality observations and in April the recommended staffing. Believing we had the most accurate data available we projected budgeted staff for FY 1976–1977 (see Table 1). We chose to add a 1.5 factor to the suggesting staffing to provide coverage for employee orientation (important to us as we projected an increase in the number of new staff), vacation (each of our employees receives ten days after one year of employment, eight holidays, including two personal holidays) and ill time. While we felt our initial staffing projects were valid for the particular time we studied, we knew our needs might change based on projected or possible changes in patient acuity. This led us into the final project phase—establishing variable staffing and meaningful daily and monthly management reporting.

KEEPING STATISTICS

There are many methods available for keeping statistics, and we had in the past been using six different forms to give us such information as unit census, daily staffing, daily average patient care hours, vacation, illness and absence, pulling from one unit to another, utilization of outside agency help and finally a monthly average of all of the above. This has been reduced

to one form which gives us everything but the monthly totals (see Figure 2).

There are almost as many ways of utilizing the classification forms. Some hospitals have the clerk on each unit add up the total points and classify the patients by hand before sending the sheets or totals to a control staffing office. Some hospitals have full computer capabilities and are able to readily transfer the information to the computer and have results within two or three hours (maybe longer in some settings). Some have utilized programmable calculators.

We have chosen the latter route, first of all because we do not feel our clerks should be used for the task of adding up the numbers of as many as 37 patients; we do not have full inhouse computer capability (this probably will be available to us in 12 to 18 months—too long to wait) and the cost factor and turn around time is reasonable and efficient. The classification sheets arrive from the units by 9:00 A.M. and within one hour information is available to us giving total census, total and average patient type, total workload and projected staffing for four shifts, all of which can be transcribed to the daily management report.

WORK WILL CONTINUE

A year has passed since we originally began our work with the Medicus Corporation and adopted the staffing with quality assurance programs. We officially completed the

TABLE 1

Sample Projected Budgeted Staff FY 1976–1977

Unit Daily Staffing

Units/ Shift	Positions Per Shift							Patient Care				Administrative			
	HN	CH	TL	Staff	LPN	NA	Total	RN	LPN	NA	Total	HN	CH	TL	Total
2W D	1	0	3	0	5	1	10	1.8	5	1	7.8	1	0	1.2	2.2
E	0	1	1	1	5	1	9	2	5	1	8.0	0	0.0	0.4	1.0
N	0	1	0	1	4	0	6	1.4	4	0	5.4	0	0.6	0	0.6
Total	1	2	4	2	14	2	25	5.2	14	2	21.2	1	1.2	1.6	3.8
2E D	1	0	2	3	4	1	11	4.2	4	1	9.2	1	0	0.8	1.8
E	0	1	1	4	4	1	11	5	4	1	10.0	0	0.6	0.4	1.0
N	0	1	1	1	5	2	10	2	5	2	9.0	0	0.6	0.4	1.0
Total	1	2	4	9	10	4	33	11.2	10	4	29.2	1	1.2	1.6	3.8
3W D	1	0	2	0	3	1	7	1.2	3	1	5.2	1	0	0.8	1.8
E	0	1	1	2	4	1	9	3	4	1	8	0	0.6	0.4	1.0
N	0	1	0	2	3	1	7	2.4	3	1	6.4	0	0.6	0	0.6
Total	1	2	3	3	11	3	22	6.6	11	2	19.6	1	1.2	1.2	3.4
3C D	1	0	0	2	0	0	2	2.0	0	0	2	1	0	0	1.0
E	0	1	0	0	2	0	3	0.4	2	0	2.4	0	0.6	0	0.6
N	0	1	0	0	1	0	2	0.4	1	0	1.4	0	0.6	0	0.6
Total	1	2	0	2	4	0	7	2.8	4	0	5.8	1	1.2	0	1.2
3E D	1	0	2	2	4	0	9	3.2	4	0	7.2	1	0	0.8	1.8
E	0	1	1	1	3	1	7	2	3	1	6.2	0	0.6	0.4	1.0
N	0	1	0	1	5	0	7	1.4	5	0	6.4	0	0.6	0	0.6
Total	0	2	3	4	12	1	23	6.6	12	1	19.8	1	1.2	1.2	3.4

Unit Daily Staffing

Units/Shift	Positions Per Shift							Patient				Administrative			
	HN	CH	TL	Staff	LPN	NA	Total	RN	LPN	NA	Total	HN	CH	TL	Total
4W D	1	0	2	1	3	0	7	2.2	3	0	5.2	1	0	0.8	1.8
E	0	1	1	1	3	0	6	2.0	3	0	5.0	0	0.6	0.4	1.0
N	0	1	0	2	3	0	6	2.4	3	0	5.4	0	0.6	0	0.6
Total	1	2	3	4	9	0	19	6.6	1	0	15.6	1	1.2	1.2	3.4
4C D	1	0	0	4	2	0	7	4	2	0	6.0	1	0	0	1.0
E	0	1	0	3	3	0	7	3.4	3	0	6.4	0	0.6	0	1.0
N	0	1	0	4	3	0	8	4.4	3	0	7.4	0	0.6	0	0.6
Total	1	2	0	11	8	0	22	11.8	8	0	19.8	1	1.2	0	2.2
5W D	1	0	2	2	4	0	9	3.2	4	0	7.2	1	0	0.8	1.8
E	0	1	1	1	4	0	7	2	4	0	6.0	0	0.6	0.4	1.0
N	0	1	0	1	5	0	7	1.4	5	0	6.4	0	0.6	0	0.6
Total	1	2	3	4	13	0	23	6.6	13	0	19.6	1	1.2	1.2	3.4
5C D	2*	0	0	6	1	0	9	6	1	0	7.0	2*	0	0	2.0
E	0	1	0	4	1	0	6	4.4	1	0	5.4	0	0.6	0	0.6
N	0	1	0	5	1	0	7	5.4	1	0	6.4	0	0.6	0	0.6
Total	2	2	0	15	3	0	22	15.8	3	0	18.8	2	1.2	0	3.2
all units D	10	0	13	20	26	3	71	27.8	26	3	56.8	10	0	5.2	15.2
E	0	9	6	17	29	4	64	24.2	30	4	58.2	0	5.4	2.4	7.8
N	0	9	1	17	30	3	61	21.2	30	3	54.2	0	5.4	0.4	5.8
Total	10	18	20	54	85	10	196	73.2	86	10	169.2	10	10.8	8.0	28.8

*1 Assist. Head Nurse

FIGURE 2. SAMPLE DAILY ADMINISTRATIVE SURVEY FORM

Unit	Unit Census	Assigned Staff			Required Staff			Float Sent to			Staff Pulled To Unit			Staff Pulled From Unit			Illness and/or Absence			Vacations			Actual Staffing			Average Patient Type				Avg. Pt. Type	Nsg. Care Hours
		RN	LPN	NA	RN	LPN	NA	RN	LPN	NA	RN	LPN	NA	RN	LPN	NA	RN	LPN	NA	RN	LPN	NA	RN	LPN	NA	I	II	III	IV		
2E D																															
2E E																															
2E N																															
3E D																															
3E E																															
3E N																															
3C D																															
3C E																															
3C N																															
4C D																															
4C E																															
4C N																															
5C D																															
5C E																															
5C N																															
2W D																															
2W E																															
2W N																															
3W D																															
3W E																															
3W N																															

> *We officially completed the project in June of 1976 but we have never really "finished" our work, nor do I visualize that we will. The program is one which is on-going within the institution with some continued limited involvement from the consultants.*

project in June of 1976 but we have never really "finished" our work, nor do I visualize that we will. The program is one which is ongoing within the institution with some continued limited involvement from the consultants. Our management report over the year has shown us that the acuity of our patients has increased on almost every unit bringing about the daily need to add additional staff on most shifts. Therefore, as we head into another budget year, we have again contracted with Medicus to do a detailed two week review of classification, workload and goals matrix to find where changes in staffing are indicated on a long-term basis.

Quality assurance reviews are done on every unit quarterly so that we are able to determine what changes, if any, are taking place. Results are reviewed by the Division of Staff

Development and inservice programs are planned on the unit level in an effort to strengthen areas of weakness as well as improve in those areas where we are strong.

We have utilized a float pool very effectively allowing us to have a flexibility within our staff each shift with limited pulling from unit to unit and limited utilization of agency help. Until acuity levels became so high and the census in ICU began running more than 100 percent, we did not use agency staff for a total of six months.

We have found that there is not the need to have a professional person doing the day to day staffing; this is done by a staffing assistant who has learned to interpret the data and assign staff as needed. Staffing assistants only seek the assistance of a nursing coordinator or head nurse when they are not able to solve a staffing problem.

It has also been apparent to us that Medicus feels the program should not be stagnant. They are continuously looking for ways to improve the methodology. As they find a better way, it is shared with us so that we too may continue to advance.

Staffing for quality patient care continues to be the concern of nursing administration in our institution. We feel we have found a method which will help us reach that goal.

REFERENCE

1. Sanders, E. J., *et al. Results of Nurse Utilization and Staffing Control Methodology for Children's Hospitals* (New York: Western New York Association of Hospital Management Engineering Programs June 1970).

The Staffing Function and Management Techniques

Kay Lillesand, B.S.N.
Director of Nursing Service
St. Nicholas Hospital
Sheboygan, Wisconsin

Laura L. Mathews, B.S.N.
Director of Nursing Service
Steven Bryant Nursing Home
Milwaukee, Wisconsin

THE QUEST is on for identification of effective management of the problems inherent in the staffing function. Finding solutions is a monumental task whether the problem is related to quality, personnel utilization, or lack of effective management. Each setting is unique, and each administrator encounters different problems.

A SURVEY

In the Spring of 1974, a small number of nursing service administrators were interviewed in order to identify the problems that they perceived as being significant to the staffing function. When the data was analyzed, eight factors were found predominant in their influence on the staffing function. A review of the literature on the subject substantiated the influence of these factors:

1. Recruitment.
2. Hospital and nursing service philosophies and goals.
3. Hospital and personnel policies.

28

Finding solutions to problems inherent in the staffing function is a monumental task whether the problem is related to quality, personnel utilization, or lack of effective management. Each setting is unique.

4. Determination of personnel requirements.
5. Administrative support.
6. Incentives and job satisfaction.
7. Use of part-time and float personnel.
8. External forces.

Other findings of the survey led us to these conclusions:

- There was a tendency to confuse the staffing function with the scheduling function.
- Recruitment programs were inadequate.
- Incentives (especially related to intrinsic factors) were lacking.
- The correlation between staff development and job satisfaction was not clearly demonstrated.
- Universally there was a lack of use of established management techniques to solve staffing problems.

USING MANAGEMENT
TECHNIQUES IN STAFFING

It is this latter point—lack of use of established management techniques —that is particularly significant. We know that management is simply the process of achieving goals through the appropriate use of human resources: people. The basic management tech-

niques of *planning, organizing, implementing,* and *evaluating* are essential if work is to be accomplished and goals are to be reached. The achievement of the hospital and nursing service goals is dependent on how successfully the staffing function is managed. The results of the survey led us to believe that a conceptual model for applying management techniques to the staffing function would be helpful.

Management is simply the process of achieving goals through the appropriate use of human resources: people.

SAMPLE INTEGRATION

To more clearly understand the interrelationship of the eight influential factors pinpointed by the survey and the management process, study Figure 1. A carefully drafted outline which tracts the management process can be very beneficial in mitigating the problems associated with the staffing function. As an example, let us use the recruitment factor. An outline integrating the management process to the recruitment factor might be created along the following lines:

I. PLANNING
   1. Develop the philosophy, purpose and objectives of the recruitment programs.
   2. Develop a recruitment committee.
   3. Forecast both short-term and long-term staffing needs.

FIGURE 1. FACTORS AFFECTING STAFFING AND THE MANAGEMENT PROCESS.

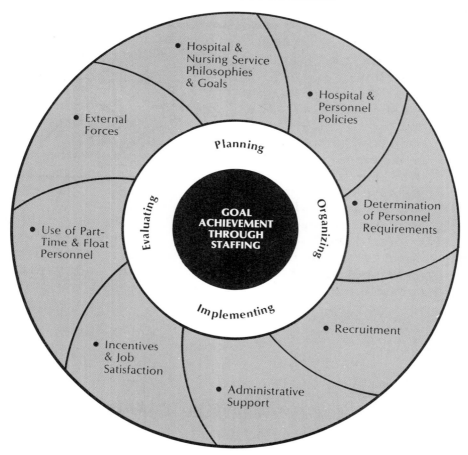

4. Determine "how" each objective will be accomplished.
5. Determine "when" each objective will be accomplished.
6. Establish a budget for the recruitment program.

II. ORGANIZING
   1. Determine recruitment policies.
   2. Establish recruitment procedures.

3. Develop job description for recruiter, including lines of authority and position requirements.
4. Establish standards of performance.

III. IMPLEMENTING
   1. Analyze resources.
   2. Select and develop staff.
   3. Delegate authority, responsibility, and accountability.

30

4. Motivate personnel—stimulate creative problem solving.
5. Initiate feedback system and give support where needed.

IV. EVALUATING
1. Effectiveness
   a. Outcomes—Did we get the staff we set out to obtain?
   b. Process—Did we recruit at the proper places? Did we use the proper methods of recruitment? Did we get an adequate return on our money?
2. Efficiency—Did we stay within the proposed budget?
3. Identify problems with existing program and replan.

As the model demonstrates, the process is cyclical in nature, for as we define areas of change we return to the planning stage and start again.

We have utilized the outline format for only a single factor—recruitment.

The process of effective management is cyclical in nature, for as we define areas of change we return to the planning stage and start again.

As the model indicates, it must be repeated for each of the eight factors. In each case, the management techniques can and must be applied for effective staffing and ultimate goal achievement.

More Effective Development for New Nurses

Alan L. Frohman, Ph.D.
Organization Consultant
Frohman Associates, Inc.
Arlington, Massachusetts

THE PROCESS of establishing the relationship between employees and supervisors is invariably stressful and often extremely frustrating for them both. The problem becomes particularly acute when the employee is a recent college graduate or an employee new to the organization. Research and experience over the past few years have confirmed the fact that employees' first 18 months are the most critical of this tenure with the organization. Valuable material and emotional resources are wasted, due to the lack of consideration of the peculiar and unique problems of new employees and the establishment of a relationship between employees and their immediate supervisors. High turnover, low motivation, low productivity, unnecessary conflict, and hence

The author wishes to acknowledge his former employer, Pugh-Roberts, Associates, Inc., Cambridge, Massachusetts. While with Pugh-Roberts, the author developed copyrighted materials that are based on and extend the concepts in this article. Some of the ideas and examples herein are drawn from his work with them.

31

32

High turnover, low motivation, low productivity, unnecessary conflict, and hence employee dissatisfaction have all been traced to mismanagement or nonmanagement of employee's early experiences with their immediate supervisors.

employee dissatisfaction have all been traced to this mismanagement or nonmanagement of employees' early experiences with their immediate supervisors.

Some years ago, managers of major industrial companies were becoming increasingly concerned with the cost and energy their companies were expending just to keep their manpower quota filled. As a consultant I began working with some of these companies, basing my approach on concepts originally developed by Edgar Schein and extended by John Kotter.[1,2]

Extra time and attention directed toward managing the initial working experience have proven extremely useful. For example, one company which hired 15 professionals a year realized a very conservative savings of over $220,000/year during their first year of focusing attention on new employees.[3] These savings resulted from: (1) reduced turnover, (2) decreased time in which it took an employee to reach "full" productivity, and (3) general increase in employee productivity. In addition, there were intangible cash savings resulting from increased employee satisfaction and

creativity, less nonproductive conflict, and greater enthusiasm.

WHAT DOES THE "EARLY EXPERIENCE" MEAN?

First, what is meant by "early experience?" It covers all those first sets of activities that an organization uses to bring new employees on board. These include recruitment, selection, hiring, orientation, the first assignment, training, introduction to the first work group (peers), and—what research and experience have unequivocally demonstrated to be the most important factor—introduction to the first supervisor. (See Figure 1.)

In a hospital setting, the most critical period—affecting productivity, learning time, attitude, and turnover—is the first six months. The

FIGURE 1. EARLY EXPERIENCE ACTIVITIES

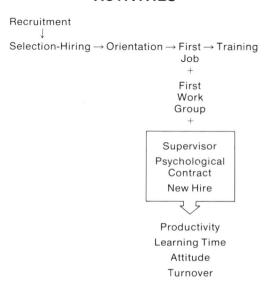

single most important factor concerning the productivity and satisfaction of staff nurses are their head nurses. Head nurses control both psychological and material rewards and are in a sense the new nurses' models, for either positive or negative reasons. To staff nurses they are, for all practical purposes, *the organization:* the hospital is not tangible to staff nurses; the people they report to are. The head nurses' attitudes, behavior, and expectations all make up the staff nurses' reality, and for these reasons the relationship between head nurses and staff nurses turns out to be the most influential in determining productivity, learning time, attitude, and turnover that staff nurses will have on their jobs. So, while the initiation period covers all of the activities mentioned above, the head-staff nurse relationship is the key in managing the entire process and improving the dimensions noted earlier.

This relationship between new employees and their first supervisor is particularly critical. New employees are permeable, in a sense; their expectations and their habits have not been so well set. They have limited previous experience to rely upon, so they come in much more open minded, bringing with them fewer behavior patterns that have to be undone. So, while one's immediate supervisor tends to be the most important factor in any job—whether the first, second, or third—it holds true to a greater extent for the first job.

One of the most critical aspects of the relationship between head nurses

One of the most critical aspects of the relationship between head nurses and staff nurses is the "psychological contract." There are two important parts to this contract: what individual employees expect to give the organization relative to what the organization expects to receive, and what the organization expects to give.

and staff nurses is what we have come to call the "psychological contract." When most employees join an organization, a contractual agreement is reached which includes reference to the organization's liabilities, responsibilities, salary, and other things that indicate what an organization expects to give its employees. Also, there is some mention of what the organization expects to receive: for example, specified hours of time a week, conformance to certain sets of rules and requirements. While this is important, it does not cover all of the key ingredients of having employees comfortable and performing well. Some of the agreements that you never find in that contract have become part of the psychological contract.

There are two important parts to this contract. The first is what individual employees expect to give the organization relative to what the organization expects to receive; and the second is what the organization expects to give. As mentioned earlier, the organization in this case is embodied in head nurses as far as the

34

staff nurses are concerned. What staff nurses expect to receive from the organization and what the organization expects to give are, from the staff nurses' perception, really what they expect to receive from their head nurses and what their head nurses expect to give.

This contract is a two-way street. Expectations generally exist, whether the participants want them to or not, and the psychological contract exists, whether people want it to or not. There is simply no way around the fact that it is likely that there are mismatches and expectations between employees and their organizations. Unless something is done to specifically deal with these differences, *inevitably* a psychological contract of mismatches develops. It is inevitable because there are factors working in society at large, and not just in the hospital situation, which cause these differences and, hence, mismatches. It is important to realize that it is not a question of whose expectations are right, and whose expectations are wrong. It is a fact that they will be different and that they need to be understood and resolved.

The match—or mismatch—between these two sets of expectations is the important, single factor influencing the relationship between head nurses and staff nurses. (See Figure 2.) Some examples follow.

1. Autonomy in schedule setting. Individual nurses may expect a certain autonomy in schedule setting. They may be willing to say to the hospital, "Yes, you may infringe upon my weekends, and yes, you may infringe upon certain amounts of my free time

FIGURE 2. PSYCHOLOGICAL CONTRACT: MATCHES AND MISMATCHES

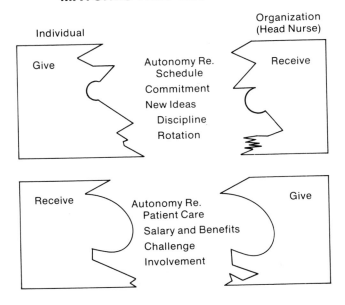

in this manner, or you may expect a certain amount of time above and beyond the normal work week." The organization also holds expectations about the amount of flexibility on the part of new employees regarding their schedules and the extent to which they can follow what the hospital requires. If what the nurses expect to give is the same as what the organization expects to receive, the expectations match satisfactorily. In a sense, the two pieces fit together, the expectations fit together, and you have the start of a sound psychological contract. On the other hand, nurses may expect to give up certain aspects of their free time, particularly with respect to rotation, and the organization may expect to receive more flexibility of schedule on the part of the new nurses (the ability to be assigned on this weekend or this holiday, or to do this or that). If the staff nurses do not expect to give up as much flexibility regarding their time assignment as the organization expects them to give up, there exists a mismatch and the making for a much less sound psychological contract.

2. Discipline. This is another example of an area where mismatches in expectations may occur. Staff nurses may expect to find a certain amount of discipline in the hospital (a certain amount of order, organization, people telling you what to do, etc.) or, on the other hand, they might expect to be allowed a certain degree of self-discipline. On one hand, they expect some direction from the hospital, the organization, and on the other hand, they expect to be able to assert themselves. The hospital may expect to receive a different amount of self-discipline from staff nurses and may not tell them what to do nearly as often as they expect. Or perhaps the hospital may expect their unquestioning obedience to their supervisors and the physicians.

As these two examples show, mismatches may begin to develop because the expectations are rarely made explicit. But they are always found in the psychological contract, either explicitly or implicitly. *These matches and mismatches in the psychological contract are the most important determinant of how effective and productive employees will be.* If serious mismatches exist, there is a much greater probability of high turnover, low productivity, and great employee dissatisfaction than if the psychological contract contains matches.

SOURCES OF DIFFERENCES

There are various reasons why there are inevitable differences in expectations between employees and head nurses. First are *generation differences.* Today, people are saying that four years' separation in age has become a generation for those under 35. A figure of 20 years, which was standard up until a few years ago, has simply changed due to the rapidity of change in society. Now, someone 21 could be a generation apart from someone 26 or 28.

Second are *institutional differences.* Even for a nurse who is simply transferring from one hospital to another,

FIGURE 3. SOURCES OF DIFFERENCES

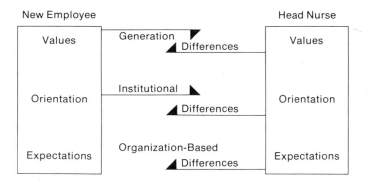

there are differences in procedures, the information organization and the like, which give rise to mismatches and expectations. (See Figure 3.)

It is important to realize that these factors are totally beyond the control of any particular individual, certainly including head nurses. These differences are inevitable. In order to get a bit more comfortable with the inevitability of externally imposed expectations, let's examine some of these in more detail.

Generation Differences[4]

1. Higher value on intellectual components. The people who come out of school more recently tend to put a much higher value on the intellectual components of their jobs. They tend to feel that challenge is equal to intellectual challenge, and that they are more intelligent than the graduate of a few years ago. It is not really important whether this is true or not; it is just a different sort of challenge in their job than someone who has been out of school for five or ten years.

2. Security secondary. Having been more accustomed to material goods and security, people today are less concerned about them and, as a result, salary and fringe benefits, those things which build security and material goods, have become secondary to other goals such as challenge, growth, and the like. This isn't to say that salary and fringes are not important, but that they simply are not enough.

3. Strong adherence to the "Protestant work ethic" declining. While it is still believed that hard work is good in and of its own sake, the notion of working 10 to 12 hours a day is less important than it was a few years ago.

4. Declining emphasis on strong adherence to authority. The schools, the church, and the family are placing decreased emphasis on obedience to authority, and the impact on the job is that head nurses can no longer rely on their position as head nurse to give them absolute authority. Staff nurses are much more likely to feel that they should be self-determining, that deci-

There is less emphasis on permanent attachment. Today's employees do not come to an organization with the expectation of working there for the rest of their lives. They come to spend a while and get what they can, and then move on.

sions should be their responsibility rather than left up to an authority to decide.

5. Less emphasis on permanent attachment. This is seen all over—in disposable diapers, in the increase in rentals of all kinds, in the divorce rate, in the rate of home and job movements, and in the nursing turnover. Today's employees do not come to an organization with the expectation of working there for the rest of their lives. They come to spend a while and get what they can, and then move on. This should not be construed in a negative sense, but more that people today are inner-directed and are less willing to sacrifice for the organization.

6. "What's in it for me?" The modern generation is asking the question "What's in it for me?" more than generations of the past. They are listening more to the drummer inside rather than the drummer out in the organization or in other groups.

Institutional Differences

There are also differences caused by different institutional backgrounds. A hospital is, obviously, its own institu-

tion, and the employees who have been members of this organization for a while learn to expect peculiarities of the organization. The new staff nurses, however, are coming directly from an educational background, such as a college or nursing school, and this background can be substantially different from that of the hospital. Several examples can illustrate this:

1. Schedule—A hospital schedule is fixed on the considerations of the patients and the medical staff and certainly tends to be more rigid than that found in an academic environment (generally a schedule that is fixed after consideration of the faculty and individual students' requirements).

2. Problems—The problems encountered in the hospital are those of the "real world," dealing with patients. Academic problems tend to be much more education-oriented, and serve the need of teaching students in the hospital. They are neat, clean, and have *one correct answer* (so they may be graded), whereas hospital problems are rarely clear or simply structured, and they may have no absolutely correct answer.

3. Supervision—In a hospital setting, the whole question of supervision takes on a much different and, many times, quite new dimension. In the academic setting, nursing students might have viewed their professor as their supervisor. However, this turns out to be very little like the reality of head nurses. Head nurses do not assign problem sets; they assign "real-

38 world" problems. They do not exist for the primary purpose of helping new staff nurses learn. The whole problem of having to work with a supervisor rather than with a professor is a new one. In the academic environment, it is relatively easy to drop a course and hence to switch supervisors; this is much more difficult in a hospital setting. The new nurses must learn to get along with the head nurses on a day-to-day basis.

4. Evaluation and Feedback—This turns out to be a very new experience, as evaluation and feedback in the hospital setting are considerably different from the same processes in the academic setting. One is not evaluated in the hospital on the ability to turn in good "paper" problems, and the types of feedback one gets tend to be considerably less structured and varied than in the academic setting. Feedback is much more individual than comparative—in a hospital setting, individual staff nurses rarely know how they are doing relative to the rest of the staff.

5. Promotion—Promotion also is a relatively new experience for new staff nurses. In school, promotion occured once every 12 months. As long as students did better than failure, they passed the course and got promoted. In a working environment, the whole question of promotion and tangible rewards takes on an entirely new meaning and dimension; it occurs much less frequently and is based on entirely different criteria.

Organization-Based Differences

The next class of differences that contribute to mismatches are organization-based differences. These differences refer to the types of steps and processes that an organization goes through in hiring new employees. The first step is usually recruiting. Typically, at this stage the organization and prospective employees don't engage in any frank exchange. Applicants try to impress the organization with their ability and skills, and the organization tries to appear in the best light possible, usually telling only the positive things about the job and working in that organization. As a result of this, unrealistically high expectations on the part of both the organization and new employees are usually set. After several months on the job, these unrealistic expectations, then unfilled, result in disappointment, usually more so on the part of the new employees who have not gone through this experience before. The organization has typically seen this process and understands that superstars may not shine as brightly after the first few months on the job.

The second step is screening. Here, the organization usually does little to try to effect a systematic match between the requirements of the job and the skills and characteristics of the candidate. Organizations usually look for the "best" candidate, regardless of whether the candidate is actually overqualified for the job. As a result, overqualified candidates become bored by their jobs. Other candidates, selected as the "best" candidates, are unequipped to handle important aspects of their jobs because they were not selected on the basis of those skills.

Following these mismatches of skills and expectations, head nurses often further contribute to the problems of new nurses. They are very busy with a job that is more than "full-time," without worrying about the anxieties and expectations of a new employee. Thus they may ignore "little" problems that seem minor to them, and they will keep recurring. Eventually these little problems become major, and they are emotionally draining for both the head nurses and the new employees. Their working relationship deteriorates, as the new nurses become disappointed with their jobs and the head nurses with the performance of the new nurses. By this time the underlying problem of mismatches is probably so curried in an avalanche of symptoms that it is very difficult to resurrect an effective relationship without a great deal of effort and energy.

The new nurses' first assignments

The purpose of the first assignment is to help the new nurses learn about their job and how to get things done. If they do not receive instruction and guidance from their head nurses, or if they are not given enough learning time, their first assignments will not be satisfactory.

may also pose a problem. The purpose of the first assignment is to help the new nurses learn about their job and how to get things done. If they do not receive instruction and guidance from their head nurses, if they are not given enough learning time, their first assignments will not be satisfactory. The results of poor first assignments are excessive start-up time and poor mastery of the job. Because they weren't given the time to work problems through slowly, the new nurses may take too long doing some of the basic routines that are expected of them, and they may not really be able to "get a handle" on how to carry out a particular procedure or handle a particular sort of patient.

These three sources of differences—generation-based, institution-based, and organization-based—plus others result in differences in values, orientation, and, probably most important, expectations, and are the prime cause of mismatches in the psychological contract between new nurses and their head nurses.

CLASSES OF EXPECTATIONS

There are two classes of expectations: *core* and *noncore*. Core expectations are uncompromisable. They are ground rules necessary for an organization to retain employees, or for employees to want to stay in an organization. If they are unmet, the employees will feel that their basic self-images are in jeopardy.

Examples of core expectations for

40

staff nurses might be autonomy and the challenge of new situations. Core expectations for the organization which might impinge on the staff nurses' expectations are (1) the ability to set employees' work schedules, and (2) the ability to deliver competent nursing care.

Noncore expectations, on the other hand, are compromisable and flexible. The employee or the organization may want something, but not "need it to survive." Examples of this for the staff nurse might be dress—pantsuit vs. dress uniform, color of uniform, or schedule. These same issues will probably tend to be noncore issues for the organization.

The important point to be made is that core and noncore expectations are self-defined. Staff nurses determine what is core and noncore for them for their past experiences. Only the individual nurses make the decisions. The hospital has absolutely no control over it. The hospital and the head nurses, on the other hand, determine what is

core and noncore for them, and the staff nurses have virtually nothing to say about that decision.

Resolving Core and Noncore Differences

How do we begin to resolve core and noncore differences? The four cells of the matrix in Figure 4 show the four possible interfaces between the organization's expectations and the employees' expectations.[6]

In the first cell, both the employee's and the organization's expectations are noncore. The easiest way to resolve these differences is to form an explicit agreement about behavior. For example, the hospital might say, "You may wear either a dress or pantsuit, but the color must be white." The staff nurse might say, "Well, I prefer to wear a pantsuit rather than a dress, but I don't care about the color."

In the second cell, an expectation is core to the hospital and noncore to the staff nurses. In this case, the em-

FIGURE 4. RESOLVING CORE AND NONCORE DIFFERENCES

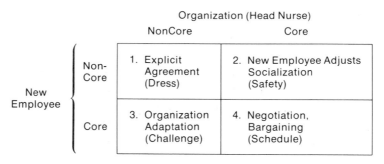

| | | Organization (Head Nurse) | |
		NonCore	Core
New Employee	Non-Core	1. Explicit Agreement (Dress)	2. New Employee Adjusts Socialization (Safety)
	Core	3. Organization Adaptation (Challenge)	4. Negotiation, Bargaining (Schedule)

1, 2, 3: Differences Are Reconcilable.
4: Differences Are Not Reconcilable.

ployees must adapt to the organization through socialization. They adapt and conform to the expectations of the organization. For example, a hospital may have a prescribed routine for giving medication. The staff nurses will be willing to follow this routine, even though they may believe that a different way is better, because the issue is noncore for them.

In the third cell, an expectation is core to the staff nurses and not to the organization. This situation is not recognized by many organizations. An example of this may be staff nurses who require an exceptional amount of challenge in their daily jobs. The hospital, through the head nurses, must adapt and offer increasingly challenging assignments to the staff nurses.

In the three cells discussed, differences were reconcilable, and at least one dimension in each cell is noncore. But in the fourth cell, there is a difference in core expectations for both parties. In the face of these "irreconcilable" differences, a process of continual negotiation, bargaining, and management needs to be undertaken. It is important to realize that differences in core expectations do not mean that the relationship must be terminated. They simply mean that the conflict that results from these differences must be constantly managed. This process can be very painful and, if not handled correctly, very energy-consuming. At the same time, it can turn out to be very rewarding for both parties.

The management of newly employed nurses' early experiences with their immediate supervisors is crucial to efficient, cost-effective staffing. In order to create a sound psychological contract between new staff nurses and their head nurses, both must clarify their expectations and explicitly communicate them to each other. Mismanagement of mismatched core expectations could lead to overconformity to the hospital's rules—"invisible employees" or "dead wood." Or it could lead to rebellion—individuals expending a great deal of energy rebelling against the hospital's expectations. Management of the differences, however, establishes a psychological contract between the individual and the organization—the committed, creative individual is able to work within the organization to accomplish the goals of both.

42

REFERENCES

1. Schein, E. H. "How to Break in the College Graduate." *Harvard Business Review* 42:6 (November–December 1964) p. 68–76.
2. Kotter, J. P. "The Psychological Contract: Managing the Joining-Up Process." *California Management Review* 15:3 (Spring 1973) p. 91–99.
3. Kotter, J. P. "Managing the Joining-Up Process." *Personnel* 49:4 (July/August 1972).
4. See Toffler, A. *Future Shock* (Random House 1970) for a thorough discussion of the differences.
5. Anthony G. Athos penetratingly examined these differences in companies in "From Campus . . . to Company . . . to Company," *Journal of College Placement* 23:12 (December 1963).
6. In "The Individual, the Organization, and the Career: A Conceptual Scheme," *Journal of Applied Behavioral Science* 7:4 (1971), Schein carries this conceptual approach he developed much further.

NAQ Forum: Staffing

MOBILIZING HUMAN RESOURCES

Eugene J. Smith, R.N., M.P.H. *Field Representative, Joint Commission on Accreditation of Hospitals, Adjunct Associate Professor, College of Nursing, University of North Carolina at Charlotte, and*

Vera F. Smith, R.N., M.S.M. *Associate Professor, Nursing, Director of Continuing Education in Nursing, University of North Carolina at Charlotte:*

The goal of that person delegated the responsibility of administrative nursing is service. The primary role of the nurse administrator is to coordinate those activities of people rendering service to others. Effective administrators not only set goals based on present needs but visualize the creative utilization of the people involved in attaining future goals. The term administrator is used to describe any professional leadership responsibility under whatever title is given this function in administrative or middle management levels in the hospital setting. Utilization involves a data bank of information about personnel and

44

patient needs and matching the two with continuing skill and understanding.

Many fundamental management principles are inherent in effective utilization of the human resources and abilities of nursing team members. The establishment of criteria for the quality of care is the first step in attaining the goal of optimal service. Each nurse administrator must audit the abilities of the "team" members. The basis of this audit should be clear, meaningful but flexible job descriptions. Information about in-service programs including orientation and other ongoing on-the-job training programs should be available to the nurse administrator. In addition to this the nurse administrator's portfolio of knowledge should include the predicted beginning competencies of graduates of the various professional and technical education programs which provide the personnel for the nursing department.

Nursing administration has the responsibility for staff development which should include management concepts for those nurses coordinating the nursing team. Barriers to effective utilization including resistance to change can be avoided through the internalization of roles reinforced by continuing education. This experience not only fosters greater self-actualization but new attitudes toward various team members who have in the past been poorly utilized.

Criteria for care once established should be reviewed and assessed frequently not only in light of quality assurance but also as it is related to changing practice. Those concerned with patient care must also take into consideration the changing expectations of society as it is reflected in patient and significant other expectation. Criteria of

care are influenced by colleague and community expectations including physicians, other health team members and faculty of the educational programs utilizing the hospital for clinical laboratory experience.

In addition to knowledge of institutional criteria, audit of the abilities of nursing staff members, numbers of personnel available and work schedules, nursing administration should have patient data which evaluates the patient population need for skilled nursing care. Innovative nursing administrators urge other administrative colleagues and physicians to experiment with non-traditional admission policies not related to diagnosis, sex or age. In a large hospital with many acutely ill patients data should be collected on nursing care needs of patient populations of given units on a 24-hour basis for several days to evaluate the staffing needs and adequacy of present systems in coping with these needs. Nursing administrators should have input into time of admission and clustering of patients in relation to skilled staff.

Automation has been initiated in many hospitals with much involvement of nursing staff. Some beneficial effects anticipated are:

1. Patient care will be upgraded as a result of a critical analysis of the job to be done through a detailed description of tasks. This information should lead to more meaningful patient care plans, better communication among team members providing care and clearer assignments.

2. Head nurses or team leaders will be freed from those various tasks which have relegated them to desk-bound spectator roles, allowing

them to relate to patients in a more effective way and giving them time to plan for care, direct the activities of team members giving care and observe the results of their efforts.

3. Evaluation of staff abilities and performance should be simplified through the use of the "incident" technique and study of performance in relation to assignments. More data for reports should be immediately available.

4. Through utilization of professional nurses' intellectual skills of decision making and judgment, there should be manifested a clearer congruency between the "ideal" and actual role of the professional nurse.

5. Clinical research in nursing should be increased as automation makes data available. New patterns of care and new modes of scientific nursing intervention should result from new technological devices.

It is inherent in the impact of new technological changes on leadership roles that carefully planned comprehensive inservice programs should be designed to prepare nurse administrators to function effectively. With knowledge and involvement resistance to change is minimized. Problems in the past were generated by the expectation by nurse administrators to assume roles for which they were totally unprepared educationally based on a decision-making process in which there was no nursing participation. Nothing sells a new concept or methodology like success. Experimental designs in staffing or new modalities of patient care should be tested and evaluated by willing team members. Creativity in all staff members should be fostered.

Vertical mobility is still the prime source of upward mobility in nursing. In our democratic society this is an expected fundamental right. Meaningful process evaluations of staff based on clearly defined competencies should be utilized to identify administrative potential providing an avenue for advancement.

Nurse administrators have other evaluation tools in addition to process evaluation. These include environmental data, retrospective audit of records and consumer evaluations.

High turnover rates and high incidence of absenteeism are excellent indices of poor utilization of staff and job dissatisfaction. Nurse administrators must take an objective searching look at the turnover rate of the agency. Turnover of staff has a negative economic impact on a hospital's budget when translated into terms of dollars and cents. Although no actual formula has been developed to evaluate this cost, inherent in it are staff recruitment, orientation, educational programs, loss of employee time during this period, as well as the paper work generated by new employees. Terminal interviews uncover covert reasons for resignations that do not appear on the written resignation.

Hospital nursing administrators must realize that individual needs are influenced by education, ideals and values. The higher on the professional ladder the employee is situated the greater the need for self-actualization. This is the basic appeal on those programs initiating primary nursing concepts. This milieu provides the nurse with an opportunity to function more independently, giving more freedom to utilize judgment, creativity and teaching skills.

46   As the practice of nursing is changed due to demographic and technological changes, new patient sophistication, new concepts of their roles by their professional team members and new members of their nursing teams, nurses have been cast into new roles as coordinators of the services rendered to patients. This role moves them into line supervision in which they must make meaningful decisions about patient care based on scientific knowledge and utilizing their judgment about the kinds of nursing interventions appropriate to meet individual patient needs. This further intensifies their need for educational programs that will support them in this role so that they will have (1) knowledge of the abilities and limitations of each individual member of their teams, (2) knowledge of principles of assignment and, (3) flexibility to meet changing employee schedules and patient needs. Most important they must constantly appraise the changing needs of their patients being aware of the stages they are in, whether (1) the health maintenance or health attainment stage, (2) increased risk stage, (3) early detection stage, (4) clinical stage, or (5) rehabilitative stage. Evaluating the ability of their staffs and the present and projected needs of their patients leads to better staff utilization, nursing team cohesiveness and job satisfaction as well as improved patient care quality.

    Not only is an intensive inservice program necessary to orient head nurses to their roles, but it is also necessary to initiate a new public relations program to introduce the physician, the hospital administrator and the public to the head nurses's new roles. Administrative and professional personnel are the keys to effective and efficient utilization of all nursing resources in any given institution.

    Programs should be studied in other institutions, in other industries and in other disciplines. Ideas which lend promise for effectiveness in your institution should be tried, adapted to your institution's needs, evaluated and revised. All existing programs should be evaluated periodically through questionnaires, performance evaluations or whatever evaluation tools found most effective in your institution. Don't be satisfied with "status quo." Tomorrow is here and there are new groups of learners with different educational needs, new technological changes, new patient sophistication and expectations, new problems in interpersonal relationships and the continuing problem of fewer skilled workers to care for greater numbers of patients. Is your program flexible enough and dynamic enough to meet these new needs? Your employees will let you know. Why not ask them?

    Much has been written about the hospital triad and the position in which nurses find themselves attempting to establish improved nursing practice. We need to tell them like it is, to define our present role, to shed past meaningless postures and to innovate change where it is needed. When this is done, greater job satisfaction will lead to a new therapeutic milieu in which all nursing team members are utilized in light of their ability.

CRITICAL CONSIDERATIONS FROM THE PERSPECTIVE OF A NURSING ADMINISTRATOR

Vernice Ferguson, R.N., M.S., F.A.A.N., *Chief, Nursing Department, Department of Health, Education and*

Welfare, Public Health Service, National Institutes of Health, Bethesda, Maryland:

The public demands accountability for responsive and responsible services rendered by competent health care professionals. Increasingly, the nursing profession is assuming this charge in its own right. Quality assurance programs and peer review emerge as mechanisms to assure that the public is served and the practitioner is worthy of the public's trust. New modalities of care including the advent of primary nursing and the all-professional nursing staff have appeared and with it, greater provider and consumer satisfaction. The "fee-for-service" concept and independent nursing practice demand more deliberate thought and, for many, new directions in staffing for nursing services.

There are impediments to creative and dynamic nursing care. Nursing must overcome them if we are to make a meaningful impact on health care in this era of the collective. When we consider the cost of preparing nurses for practice and the compensation received for nursing services rendered at the work site, it is abundantly clear that nurses owe their public reliable and competent services. Traditional hierarchical organizations in which edicts flow down to those providing direct nursing care are discovering that in-depth analysis and research are needed to support or refute this organization for providing nursing care and the appropriate utilization of staff in the most cost effective and professionally responsible manner.

The effective director of nursing is critical as decision maker, explicator, facilitator and change agent for nursing practice. Too often in our organizations we implement programs without the planning which must precede the change process and the evaluation which will be required on a continuum. I consider the leadership of the director of nursing crucial in establishing and maintaining the authority and accountability of nursing for its practice and fostering a climate conducive to the full participation of the nursing staff in planning, implementing and evaluating care. It would be naive, however, to assume that achieving these goals will occur in an insular nursing department. Establishing a communications network and planning strategically beyond the nursing department are required. The director of nursing has the responsibility to initiate and sustain these efforts.

Before a plan for staffing is effected the organizational structure and climate in which nursing is practiced require study and reordering if indicated. Does the organizational structure impede or facilitate a participatory and dynamic practice? Where in the organization's structure is the nursing department and how is nursing represented in policy making and evaluation of the institution's mission? What continuing education efforts and support systems are evident which support a collegial practice and review of that practice among peers?

As directors of nursing proceed to explicate, facilitate and promote change in establishing and sustaining nursing's authority and accountability for its practice they find it increasingly difficult to address nursing's unique contribution to patient care without ambiguity. Planning would be more deliberate and assured if this could be achieved, yet in the real world of practice just as constant change

48

must be considered, so too must ambiguity and flexibility be accommodated.

The nursing profession must hasten to agree on a definition of nursing, its practice and preparation for that practice. Should nurses manage the patient care environment, manage patient care, give patient care or attend to combinations thereof? We cannot address the elimination of non-nursing activities and the role of nurses with reasonable clarity and consistency until we have defined what nursing is and what nursing does. To assist us in this definition I would suggest as a starter an intellectual exercise. Imagine that a nursing service contracted out its services. What would nursing provide? At what level? At what cost? Another useful approach often posed by this director of nursing is a series of questions which must be addressed continually as we practice in a given setting. Why is the patient/client here? What can nursing provide? How does nursing and its patient/client know that we have done it well?

Is nursing an administrative or professional service? Some directors of nursing have answered this question to their satisfaction. Is there general agreement that the nursing service director's role exists to facilitate the practice of nursing which is a professional service? If we are in agreement, the professional model requires attention. The governance of the department through its bylaws and the authority for the rendering of an essential patient/client service through admitting privileges are essential.

The director of nursing fosters and sustains a climate which encourages the full participation of the staff in planning, implementing and evaluating care. Critical to this result and the staffing required to achieve it is the budget process. It should reflect the beliefs and practices of the nursing staff as it fulfills its mission and role. These include role designations, as well as allocated positions with a planned provision of time to think, to create, to plan and evaluate, thereby assuring continued competence and improved nursing care. Directors of nursing should exert leadership in bringing to fruition planned time for scholarly endeavors, as well as relief to restore staff from the exhaustion of the daily work routine. Sabbatical leave for those in organized hospital nursing services is needed, for creative and dynamic nursing care demands the renewal of its staff. Educational pursuits, research activity and relief from the work site contribute to this renewal directed toward improved nursing practice.

The director of nursing is afforded a unique opportunity to support an incentives program for the nursing staff as recognition of a nursing practice that exceeds the established standards. What are some of the considerations? Are there rewards and sanctions within the nursing domain to encourage an authoritative and accountable practice? Does the incentives program suggest to the newcomer, as well as the long established employee, that it is rewarding to be a part of the organization's nursing staff? Is it acceptable to take risks? Is the full professional role recognized and supported? Is clinical practice rewarded? Is nursing research valued? Is the continual acquisition of knowledge and its application to practice expected and accommodated? Is knowing, as well as doing, rewarded?

Staffing for nursing services aimed toward recruitment without due consideration for retention is meaningless. The director of nursing is cognizant of the many critical considerations that are required to implement and sustain a responsive staffing program. These dimensions require astute attention if nursing is to achieve its mission well in advance of the sophisticated and often ritualistic mechanisms associated with staffing for nursing care.

Centralized Scheduling: Is It Worth the Effort?

Gloria Swanberg, R.N., M.N.A.
Principal Consultant

Eunice Lawrenz Smith, R.N., B.S.N.E.
Associate Consultant
Herman Smith Associates
Hospital Consultants
Hinsdale, Illinois

FEW ACTIVITIES are more complex than scheduling nursing personnel for patient care units—frequently three or more skill levels on a minimum of three shifts daily, seven days a week—for patient care units that vary in size and need. The task becomes considerably more complex when employees are scheduled for every other weekend off, rotating shifts, or both. Hospital administrators—and even nursing administrators—frequently underestimate the magnitude of this task and commonly fail to recognize its importance in consistent quality of care, job satisfaction of employees, and cost containment.

In the majority of hospitals, personnel schedules are prepared by head nurses, usually without guidelines or assistance. They often perform this time-consuming activity while off duty and tend to schedule hours for

Adapted from ''Living Within Our Means'' presented at a meeting of the American Society of Nursing Service Administrators, Atlanta, November 1976.

52

full-time employees around part-time staff and special requests.

In the past ten to 15 years, many nursing service departments have attempted to centralize this activity and, not infrequently, have been disappointed to find problems seeming to increase rather than decrease. However, in working with well over 150 hospitals, we have become convinced that the problems often attributed to centralization are long-standing organizational and management problems, previously unrecognized and subsequently revealed by the new scheduling system. The nursing administrator who focuses on

> *The nursing administrator who focuses on solving problems rather than abandoning the system is likely to find that the total organization is strengthened and the advantages of centralized scheduling outweigh the disadvantages.*

solving those problems rather than abandoning the system is likely to find that the total organization is strengthened and the advantages of centralized scheduling outweigh the disadvantages.

ADVANTAGES OF CENTRALIZED SCHEDULING

Centralized scheduling has two major advantages:

- **Fairness for all employees.** Consistent, impartial, and objec-

tive application of policies, fair labor standards provisions, and contracts are facilitated.

- **Opportunities for cost containment by better use of resources.** These often include a reduction of "peaks and valleys" with an overall reduction in nursing hours per patient day, overtime, or both; fewer supervisory hours spent in scheduling activities; and a more effective monitoring system.

Those who favor scheduling at the unit level usually identify "more individualized treatment of employees" as its chief advantage. We have found, however, *some* employees receive more individualized treatment at the expense of others. Those who regularly make special requests may, in effect, plan their own schedules, making it necessary to assign remaining hours to the less vocal members of the staff. Schedules are also used as a part of the punishment/reward system of the scheduler, sometimes inadvertently.

CASE REPORT

The situation in Hospital X illustrates a common sequence of events. The nursing administrator decided centralization of scheduling was the best way to get the job done. She set the date, announced the decision to the head nurses, promoted a ward secretary to the new position of scheduling secretary, and added a desk in the corner of the supervisors' office for her to begin the job. Head nurses were instructed to turn over information on staffing for their units, and each deposited an envelope on the scheduling secretary's desk, indicating they were glad to comply, with comments such as, "You're welcome to take over this mess." The envelopes contained numerous special instructions on scraps of paper, for example, "can never work Friday evening," "bowls on Tuesdays," "class Wednesday evenings for the next six weeks," "babysitter has Monday off," "Jane and Susan should not be scheduled to work together," and so on and so forth.

At a head nurse meeting following the publication of the first two schedules, the nursing administrator was bombarded with complaints about the scheduling secretary:

- She doesn't understand our people as individuals.
- She schedules people to come on at 7 A.M. after working the evening before so that they have less than eight hours of sleep or call in ill.
- Sometimes nurses work eight days in a row.
- I told her that Jane and Susan should never work the same shift. They have already been scheduled together twice, and I've had to change their hours because neither is strong enough to take charge.
- I called and asked for more help yesterday when we were really swamped, and she said that we were not budgeted for more staff. I resent this from her!

- I thought that we were going to have *less* work; it seems like *more*.
- She told me to talk to Shirley because of her frequent tardiness. I told her that she had the facts and should do it herself.

After the meeting, the nursing administrator discussed the situation with the scheduling secretary and found the secretary's frustration to exceed that of the head nurses.

In this situation, and in most situations when centralized scheduling fails, the complaints and frustrations could be avoided or greatly reduced with adequate planning and clear identification of line and staff responsibilities for staffing/scheduling activities.

PLANNING

Planning for centralized scheduling must include careful determination of

---

Planning for centralized scheduling must include careful determination of the staffing needs of the scheduling office, qualifications for the positions, adequate space and privacy to concentrate on the job.

---

the staffing needs of the scheduling office, qualifications for the positions, adequate space and privacy to concentrate on the job. However, scheduling—whether centralized or decentralized—is only one part of the total staffing program, and sound planning for all aspects of the program

54

is essential for the success of any part of it.

A master staffing pattern for each unit that specifies the number of employees by category and shift for an average daily workload is a basic requirement. A plan for changes in the allocation of staff for variances in the workload should be established. The master pattern becomes the basis for projecting the personnel budget.

Head Nurse Participation

Head nurses should be held accountable for personnel expenditures over which they have control. To do so, they *must participate actively* in determining the staffing needs for their individual units and *must understand fully* the method of projecting full-time equivalents and calculating nursing hours per patient day (actual hours worked and total paid). Employees in staff departments with expertise in collecting and reporting statistics should furnish regular, timely, brief reports to their head nurses for quick reference in monitoring actual hours compared to budgeted hours. Computer reports, designed primarily for use by the financial department with voluminous information of little or no value to head nurses, are provided in some hospitals, but are seldom useful in the effective management of the nursing unit.

Policy Determinations

A second basic requirement for a successful scheduling system—centralized or decentralized—is clearly defined and understood scheduling policies. Without specific policies for scheduling employees in the nursing department as an adjunct to personnel policies that apply to all hospital employees, consistent and equitable treatment of nursing staff is impossible. Typically, policies relate to approved shifts, number of weekends off, identification of weekend days for the night shift, minimum and maximum consecutive workdays, time lapse between shifts if personnel rotate, and the scheduling of holidays and vacations. Policies for both full-time and part-time employees are delineated.

Head nurses who have participated actively in determining the staffing needs, have projected the personnel budget for their units and have meaningful, timely information regarding achievement of budgetary goals can and will be accountable for personnel expenditures over which they have control. If they have the authority to prepare and control their budgets, understand and support the schedul-

If head nurses have the authority to prepare and control their budgets, understand and support the scheduling policies, and have an opportunity for effective communication with the scheduler for their units, they will have little hesitancy to relinquish responsibility for scheduling personnel.

ing policies, and have an opportunity for effective communication with the scheduler for their units, they will have little hesitancy to relinquish responsibility for scheduling personnel.

LINE AND STAFF ACCOUNTABILITY

Recent years have seen an expansion of staff departments and positions in hospitals. Examples are the departments of personnel, management engineering, finance, staff education, and purchasing. Often, the purpose and authority of these staff departments/positions have not been clearly defined. Confusion about responsibility and authority results in staff personnel making decisions in areas where line managers are accountable.

Line positions in the nursing department are supervisory (management positions at the level of head nurse and above); these nurses are accountable for nursing care of patients on specified units or services. When scheduling is centralized, the employees in the scheduling office are in a staff relationship with management personnel in the nursing department.

The relationship between staff and line roles is described well in *Nursing Administration: Theory for Practice with a Systems Approach,* by Arndt and Huckabay:

. . . The simplest way to clarify the authority relationship between staff and line . . . is in terms of accountability. In any organizational relationship, the unit or person held accountable for the specified result has authority to make the necessary decision. Line . . . connotes authority to take action . . . to make decisions.

Staff . . . connotes the unit, or units that supply facts and information that will enable the accountable administrator to make the best decision.

Staff supplies services designed to help the line administrator achieve the best results, but the staff cannot impose its judgment or its service on the administrator with line authority.

. . . When the question of authority is at issue, it is the accountability for results that determines where the line authority resides.[1]

Staff personnel are best used when several operating units are well coordinated; expertness, adequate attention, and objectivity will increase effectiveness; line managers are likely to be loaded to capacity; and assignment has a specialized nature. To be effective, staff personnel must have ready access to information and be consulted regularly by line managers.

Line Functions in Staffing/Scheduling

In staffing and scheduling, centralized or other, it is essential for the nurses in management positions to be responsible for the following line functions:

1. Establish and control the personnel budget.
2. Develop a master staffing pattern based on patient needs and the method of assignment.
3. Develop procedures for adjustment of staff on a daily basis.

56

4. Establish requirements for each position on the staff (such as assignment to an intensive care unit or charge responsibility).
5. Develop employees to meet requirements of their positions and evaluate their performance.
6. Hire, promote, discipline, and discharge employees.

Staff Functions in Staffing/Scheduling

The staff functions for which the central scheduling office is responsible are the following:

1. Gather facts and prepare reports for line personnel to facilitate budgeting.
2. Schedule employees according to policies in staffing patterns established by line personnel.
3. Implement procedures for reallocation of staff to meet daily needs; consult immediate superior when demand exceeds supply.
4. Implement procedures for position control.
5. Maintain records needed by line managers for evaluation (regarding absenteeism for example).
6. Maintain effective communications with appropriate departments, such as personnel and payroll.

When the difference between line and staff functions is not understood, both by head nurses and by employees in the scheduling office, conflict may arise.

When the difference between line and staff functions is not understood, both by head nurses and by employees in the scheduling office, conflict may arise. The head nurses may feel they have lost authority, particularly when a question arises regarding the adequacy of the staff on their units to meet current needs. When employees in the scheduling office are not clear regarding their responsibilities and authority, they may feel totally responsible for controlling the budget, and their reactions may be extreme—either too rigid, alienating line personnel and impeding effective nursing, or too accommodating, attempting to do everything anyone requests.

FEASIBILITY

As with any major change, no centralized scheduling system, no matter how well planned, can totally avoid problems during the implementation phase. These problems may appear to be greater than those existing prior to the change, and there may be a temptation to abandon the program.

We believe that an effective centralized scheduling system is feasible and has extensive benefits for the total nursing service. The system will work if these guidelines are followed:

- A realistic personnel budget based on master staffing patterns and procedures to accommodate variations in workload is developed with active participation of head nurses;

- Scheduling policies are established, publicized, and enforced;
- Scheduling personnel are carefully selected and oriented to meet the specified needs of the scheduling program;
- Head nurses have opportunities for frequent, meaningful communication with the scheduling staff;
- Line and staff relationships are clearly delineated and understood.

As with implementation of any other far-reaching program, a commitment on the part of administration is essential. Head nurses can and should be held accountable for the quality and cost of nursing care. To do so, they need appropriate resources, including strong staff support. Centralized scheduling is an excellent way to provide support and, in answer to the question posed in the title of this article, is well worth the effort.

REFERENCE

1. Arndt, C., and Huckabay, L.M.D. *Nursing Administration: Theory for Practice with a Systems Approach* (St. Louis: C.V. Mosby Co. 1975).

Decentralization and Staffing

Ruth Barney Fine, R.N., M.N., F.A.A.N.
Associate Professor
Community Health Care Systems
School of Nursing
University of Washington
Seattle, Washington

MANY OF THE principles of organization and administration used by nursing service directors come from other disciplines such as business. The idea of matrix organization as decentralization of authority and responsibility originated in the airplane manufacturing industry and grew from many of the same conditions and needs faced by nursing directors who operate nursing departments in complex institutions.

Examination of the origin of ideas and concepts aides in the development of relationships between ideas. Such relationships help reduce the complexity of and aid in the utilization of the concepts in novel situations. The commonalities in industry and hospitals are relative to complexity, technology, environment, and uncertainty. Generalizations drawn from these relationships apply to the need for decentralization in a nursing department. The weaknesses of decentralization and application of in-

60

> *The commonalities in industry and hospitals are relative to complexity, technology, environment, and uncertainty. Generalizations drawn from these relationships apply to the need for decentralization in a nursing department.*

dustry's solutions to those weaknesses may be applied to nursing.

Three major reasons led industries to research and implement the matrix organization:

1. The increasing complexity of organizations characterized by turbulent environments.
2. The intensive technology prevalent in complex organizations.
3. The problems of dealing with uncertainty and ambiguity in the communication and decision-making structure of complex institutions.

Technology is defined as the ensemble of practice by which one uses available resources to achieve goals, and refers to the performance of certain tasks or activities. Technology is more than a machine, although there may quite likely be an interaction between the machine side of technology and specialized technique (knowledge). Technology refers to the environment in which we live; it also consists of skills of body and brain.[1]

Industries have used three main approaches to mediate uncertainty:

1. Broaden the decision-making base by decentralization of technical decision making.
2. Retain the hierarchical structure for the purposes of action decisions, formation of tactics, strategies, long-term planning and ideology.
3. Increase feedback mechanisms for control.

What are the relationships between these concepts and nursing service organizations?

TURBULENT ENVIRONMENT AND INTENSIVE TECHNOLOGY

Complex organizations are those organizations in which there are many variables: many happenings which are occurring at once and which are more than we can comprehend at one time. These happenings, or events, are subject to influences which we cannot control. Although we try to predict the happening and plan for control, we often do not have adequate information to forecast events with any degree of certainty. The influence of the external environment adds to the uncertainty in problem solving.

An Illustration

To illustrate this, observe the events in a medical center. The traditional role of an administrative supervisor in a large complex organization is to receive information, and plan for meeting the events predicted in order to offer a rational plan to the personnel on the nursing unit. This managerial role, as characterized by Thompson, is the mediation between the technical and institutional levels.[2] The supervisor attempts to eliminate as much uncertainty as possible. For example, a supervisor on the evening shift receives a call from the admitting clerk informing her that a call has been received from a resident telling her that he has accepted a patient who is in acute renal failure as a result of a car accident. The patient had been trapped in a car which had gone over an embankment. The car had been undetected for several days. The supervisor now must try to get more information from the resident. Would the patient need immediate operating room care for other injuries, recovery room care, surgical intensive care, or would the patient need immediate dialysis?

Each of the problems would need different arrangements for already scarce resources and as the shift progressed into the night, the resources would become even more scarce. The resident cannot furnish the information because he has no more information than that which he gave to the admitting clerk. In the meantime, the supervisor feels she must make contingency plans for this patient as well as other emergencies which are arising.

Some of the emergencies will use the resources as planned; others may not. The supervisor may have instituted elaborate plans to meet the emergency of the dialysis patient only to find that the patient expired en route; or that the patient needs immediate surgery for a head injury and the problem of kidney failure will have to wait. At the same time, other events are occurring which were not predicted and for which the supervisor cannot make rational plans or mediate between the incoming patient problems and the technical problems at the nursing unit level.

Cooperation Between Organizations

This uncertainty in the environment is a characteristic of turbulent field environments. Kingdon outlines the characteristics of turbulent field environments as requiring adjustments between organizations which are not alike but whose activities are, in general, positively correlated.[3] Examples might be the state patrol and the emergency room, the crippled childrens' bureau in a state and the operation of the premature center in a hospital, small referring hospitals and a large medical center, large community hospitals and extended care facilities, nursing homes, mental health agencies, halfway houses and other agencies having interactions with the complex general hospital.

Cooperation between many external agencies has increased the internal complexity of the general hospital. The hospital having a premature intensive care unit will have made interdependent arrangements with many community and regional hospitals, crippled childrens' agencies, ambulance companies, air evacuation units of military or civilian police, etc. Such arrangements require special groups within the hospital to keep the system working.

62 Similar arrangements are made for each specialty within the organization. Relationships are established between psychiatric nursing units and their halfway houses, state mental hospitals and the judicial system. Each external institution forms links with the appropriate internal specialty in a hospital. This requires different structural forms and different decision-making modalities.

Change

The second major element in the turbulent field environment as outlined by Kingdon, is the presence of change caused by new and different procedures arising from innovation, research and advanced technology.[4] Advanced or intensive technology in

---

Advanced or intensive technology in hospitals has been the major cause of change adding to the turbulent environment in which nursing is practiced.

---

hospitals has been the major cause of change adding to the turbulent environment in which nursing is practiced. The nursing areas such as nursing units, operating rooms, intensive care units, emergency rooms, burn units and all patient care areas are impacted by the intensive technologies in use in general hospitals.

DEALING WITH UNCERTAINTY BY CHANGING STRUCTURE

Technology, as defined by Kast, "has two aspects—the physical manifestation such as machinery and equipment and the accumulated knowledge concerning the means to accomplish tasks."

Different technologies require different relationship patterns. Perrow emphasizes the tendencies of organizations to match structure with technology. He has examined nonroutine technologies and structure and has drawn the conclusion that nonroutine technologies in which the production workers deal with many exceptions, need discretion and power and an open organic system in which to function.[6] On a nursing unit there are many specialities, many individuals, many occurrences which are not predictable (high uncertainty). Decision making carried out in such an environment has a high degree of risk. In addition, the task-related interactions between nurse and doctor, nurse and physical therapist, nurse and respiratory therapist, to mention a few, produce high interdependence among and between the various groups.

This interdependence creates the need for coordination at the technical level of the nursing unit. The traditional expectation that the supervisor will coordinate all activities for the unit will not work since much of the coordination needs to be done in on-the-spot discussion. For example, the admission of a patient to an intensive care unit needs to be negotiated between the nurse on the unit and the resident. The nurse needs to communicate the present needs of the patients in the unit and the resources of the staff. Negotiations need to be made about moving less critical patients out of the unit, or changing the intensity of care for others, delaying procedures for some, or changing responsibility for procedures from nurses to residents for others. These negotiations are necessary in order to accommodate the incoming patient. In addition, should any of the variables in patient care change, feedback systems between the various groups are needed for immediate coordination.

The graduation of intensive technology will determine the power structure of the organization and the method of achieving change in the organization. Many authorities have pointed out expertise as a basis of authority, among them Uddy, who stresses that the greater the amount of technical knowledge required in an organization, the greater the emphasis on expertise as a basis of legitimate authority.[7]

The establishment of nursing authority in clinical matters had its beginning in such highly technical areas as coronary care units, intensive care units, burn centers, etc. As nurses began to acquire expertise in these areas, physicians began to recognize their authority in technological matters.

Communication Is Important

Peer relationships or nearly equal relationships, developed from the communication patterns which were necessary in such highly interdependent tasks. The result of such arrangements is that the power in the hierarchical structure is diffused and becomes a part of the communication network established by the nurse and the doctor within the areas of their expertise. The matrix organization legitimizes the lateral communication network by recognizing the authority of expertise at the staff nurse level.

Auguste Compte is quoted in Aron as saying, "The way from knowledge to power is a direct road." Aron points out that from "technical rationality as manifested in science and production, there is a logical transition to the rationality of social organization, or at least some of its aspects."[8] Industry has found that conflict resolution is a major requirement of a decentralized organization. In such organizations, interaction is a built-in requirement, and each party is an expert in a specific area, hence conflict is bound to follow. The resolution of conflict in the industrial matrix model is by group problem solving, and negotiations are used for alterations in the task structure. Feedback is used for coordination of efforts.

COMPLEX ORGANIZATIONS WILL HAVE CONFLICT

Intensive technology requiring the use of many specialties and many dis-

64

ciplines requires a structure open to many inputs; consequently, such an organization will be subject to much more tension than organizations with less complex technologies. Decentralization of control and decision making necessitates a more organic philosophy of management. Openness is a requirement of a decentralized organization. Personalities of many different participants become involved in the decision making of the work groups. Emotional issues arising from the subcultural values of nursing and the subcultural values of medicine may interfere with interactions. The organic model described by Kingdon presupposes a colleague relationship in which "mutual respect, commitment to the task, and common interests in learning and in technical achievement (these) forge the effective work group."[9]

In the open or organic organization, conflict is brought into the open and handled through negotiation. Conflict handled in this way tends to test reality, initiate innovation and help in the sharpening of ideas. March and Simon list the four major processes in which organizations react to conflict: problem solving, persuasion, bargaining and politics.[10] Problem-solving and bargaining are an integral part of an intensive technological order. Explorations offered by March and Simon show that the more organizational conflict represents individuals rather than intergroup conflicts, the greater the use of problem solving and persuasion. "Conversely, the more organizational conflict represents intergroup differences, the greater the use of bargaining."[11]

Integration of tasks in a work setting is dependent upon problem solving through mutual adjustment and self-regulation, establishing contracts such as negotiated workloads, negotiating other work agreements as illustrated by timing of nurse-doctor rounds and agreements to facilitate work of each party.[12] As individuals participate in defining such tasks as well as performing their own task, the demands on the individual are much greater and commitment to the objective and goals in the patient care area are increased. Individuals in such circumstances experience role conflict. They receive pressures from two or more areas making compliance more difficult in any one area. They also have problems with role interdependence since the giving and receiving of information is essential for the performance of their roles. Because of the stresses and strains of role ambiguity, maladaptive behavior may arise.

In the open or organic organization, conflict is brought into the open and handled through negotiation. Conflict handled in this way tends to test reality, initiate innovation and help in the sharpening of ideas.

STAFF DEVELOPMENT

Most nurses on a staff level do not have adequate group development training to equip them to function in an environment where negotiation of roles is necessary and problem-solving work groups are the medium for decision making. Training in group development is essential for all members interacting in a decentralized environment. Participation training is described by Bergevin "... as an educational means for helping persons help themselves; that is helping them to learn how to learn."[13] Because of decentralization attempts to optimize relationships between individuals and groups, group development must be used. Nursing departments may spend considerable time and resources in participation training for staff nurses, but this is usually done in isolation without the other members of the group such as dietitians, social workers, residents, interns, respiratory therapists and others. The major problem here is to gather the chief role holders into participation training sessions in order to build a collaborative culture. Emotional issues between doctors and nurses need to be faced and resolved in group development sessions.

Decentralization in nursing has provided the various disciplines that comprise the membership of the nursing units who believe in and use the complementary principle. Kingdon has formulated the complementary principle and expresses it as follows: "when two individuals are given a common task, each can take into account the views of the other while simultaneously holding his own view of the task. Further, when the value of holding a reciprocal view of the common task is shared by the two individuals, there is less need for higher order mechanism of control to integrate their views so that they may regulate each other and thus act in concert. Finally, when (a) the environment in which the two find themselves is relatively complex and the outcomes of their task relationship are relatively uncertain (requiring innovation), and (b) an optimal solution representing multiple performance criteria is desired, a complementary relationship is preferred over a relationship that is principally controlled by the hierarchical manager." Kingdon continues with an extremely important point, one which needs much attention if decentralization is to work, especially in areas where nurses and doctors interact.

"The complementary relationship differs from a hierarchical relationship, or an authority relationship, inasmuch as neither participant is subordinate to the other. However, this does not mean that the two are necessarily equal. The role that each participant plays in the relationship is defined principally as a function of their shared task."[14]

The above quotations should receive considerable thought when decentralization of a nursing department is considered. The concept of "team" among professionals has not worked well since the values held by medicine are supported, in part, by society. The physician members of the "team" have tended to assume that

66

they were the captains of the team and because of this concept in some, perhaps many instances, tended to wield power in an inappropriate manner. The use of unrestrained power in a decentralized structure can be very destructive.

Decision Making

When decentralized planning is considered, all professional participants from every discipline represented should accept the premise of split decision making.

The decision making in regard to the socio-technical system on the nursing units or clinical areas is different from and somewhat separated from the decision making level at the nursing administration level. *However, each professional discipline is accountable in a hierarchical manner to the professional administrative system.* Nurses are responsible to the Director of Nursing, physicians are responsible to the Medical Director, social workers are responsible to the Director of Social Work. In this manner, there is a focus of work on consumer tasks at the lowest level of decision making. A structure is also maintained for a community of interest for professional objectives. In general, all goals and objectives for nursing as a group continue to be developed by nursing personnel in a group effort for the total department. Plans for allocation of resources, strategies for continuing development of staff as patient advocates, and implementation of new procedures and practices will continue to be developed under the leadership

of the nursing administrator. Authority regulation is associated with establishment of goals and objectives, the use of normative values inherent in a professional subculture and use of an idealogical belief system. The linkage provided by the nursing administration in providing guidance and developing the socio-technical system is very important if the organization is to be a unified whole rather than a disjointed system.

DECENTRALIZATION INCREASES NURSING POWER

The control in the socio-technical system is based on self-regulation through feedback mechanisms. If the goals of the nursing department are

> *If the goals of the nursing department are accepted by the nursing staff, the decentralized organizational structure expands the nursing power in the organization.*

accepted by the nursing staff, the decentralized organizational structure expands the nursing power in the organization. Each staff nurse then becomes an emissary for nursing and the care component is increased by each nurse.

Historically, the nursing department administrator has been highly dependent on administrative supervisors to transfer the goals and philosophies to the socio-technical levels in the institution; much has been lost in the transfer of such information. If each staff nurse developed the appropriate behaviors for self-regulation and was fully involved in the development of philosophy goals and objectives for the department so that each was fully equipped to participate as well as to produce, the power of the nursing department would be tremendously expanded. This expansion of power would be at the working level where negotiated interaction between members of various disciplines occurs and where the impact is the greatest for changes in patient care.

In summary, many of the same reasons for decentralization exist in hospital nursing departments as in industry. Certainly, tertiary hospitals are complex, have a turbulent environment and operate under intensive technologies. The need for authorized patterns of communication exists between staff nurses and other disciplines with whom they work. The recognition of the expertise of the staff nurse and the placing of technical responsibility and authority at this level is needed to unify nursing and promote the best interests of the patient.

Decentralization carried out in the proper manner can cement the relationships between the top and bottom level of the nursing organization and counteract the increasing alienation of staff nurses and nursing administrators. The mission of the department of nursing would be strengthened and the tendency of staff nurses at the unit level to disassociate from the nursing department would be reversed, since each nurse would experience nursing goal continuity and congruence.

REFERENCES

1. Kast, F. E. and Rosenzweig, J. E. *Organization and Management* (New York: McGraw-Hill Book Company 1974) p. 181.
2. Thompson, J. D. *Organizations in Action: Social Service Base of Administrative Theory* (New York: McGraw-Hill Book Company 1967).
3. Kingdon, D. R. *Matrix Organization Managing: Information Techniques* (London: Tavistock Publications, Limited 1973) p. 12.
4. *Ibid.* p. 12.
5. Kast, *Organization and Management.* p. 204.
6. Perrow, C. B. *Organizational Analysis: A Sociological View* (Belmont, California: Brooks Cole Publishing Company 1970) p. 80–85.
7. Uddy, S. H., Jr. "The Comparative Analysis of Organizations." *Handbook of Organizations.* James G. March, ed. (Chicago: Rand McNally and Company 1965) p. 678–706.
8. Aron, R. *The Industrial Society* (New York: Frederick A. Praeger 1967) p. 70.
9. Kingdon, *Matrix Organization Managing.* p. 83.
10. March, J. G. and Simon, H. A. *Organizations* (New York: John Wiley and Sons, Inc. 1958) p. 129.
11. *Ibid.* p. 130.
12. Fine, R. B. "Controlling Nurses Workload." *The American Journal of Nursing* (December, 1974) p. 2206–2207.
13. Bergevin, P. and McKinley, J. *Participation Training for Adult Education* (New York: Feffer and Simons, Inc. 1965) p. 5.
14. Kingdon, *Matrix Organization Managing.* p. 61.

Viewpoints:
Staffing A Primary Nursing Unit

Joan O'Leary, R.N., Ed.D.
Vice President

Ethel Hill, R.N.
Assistant Vice President
Nursing Service
Bayfront Medical Center
St. Petersburg, Florida

THE FIRST Nursing Service Standard of the Joint Commission on Accreditation of Hospitals (JCAH) calls for a "sufficient number of duly licensed Registered Nurses on duty at all times . . . to give patients the nursing care that requires the judgment and specialized skills of a Registered Nurse."[1]

This standard, as interpreted by the JCAH, states that the number of RNs and ancillary nursing service personnel needed for each nursing unit can be determined only by evaluating the needs of the patients and the capabilities of the nursing staff assigned to the unit. In order to meet the needs defined by the JCAH, appropriate staffing must be designated.

The staffing system discussed in this article is based on a lengthy projection of individual patients' needs for nursing time and a daily assessment of acuity.

To meet staffing needs at Bayfront Medical Center, traditional methods and those created from staff feedback were combined into a system generously laced with trial and error. Although less than scientific, it is a functional system for making management decisions in an environment in which the only semiconstant factor is the number of patient beds.

Factors influencing staffing methods vary constantly: The number of patients filling those beds changes; the difficulty of the cases on hand changes; the complexity of therapies ordered changes; and the number of staff available from the community may vary, as may the utilization of various special sectors (OR, OB, CCU), and the assignment methods used.

QUALITY OF CARE AND THE HEAD NURSE

Delivery of quality care is the goal around which staffing systems are built. The quality of care delivered is determined by the quality of the system, which is ultimately determined by the head nurse. The head nurse is responsible for evaluating staff and providing opportunities for their development.[2] Head nurses are

---

Delivery of quality care is the goal around which staffing systems are built. The quality of care delivered is determined by the quality of the system, which is ultimately determined by the head nurse.

---

the individuals most qualified to adjust the abilities and caseloads of staff nurses to meet their determination of patients' needs. When a primary nurse's caseload is too heavy, it is the head nurse who assesses what help is needed and assures that the need is met. For these reasons, the head nurse is crucial to the development and implementation of a quality staffing system.

Many variables influence a head nurse's determination of staffing needs:

1. **Age and length of employment:** Longer-employed head nurses, accustomed to status quo in perseverance on the job, might tend not to suggest new and innovative staffing guidelines. The old concept, "why rock the boat?" does have to be redirected to a new focus.

2. **The socialization process:** Freedom is often accepted slowly by longer-term employees. Often they test and retest that freedom to validate their perceptions. They may socialize slowly in this environment. Their role often must be defined and redefined.

3. **Role definition and diversity:** An informal atmosphere, a first-name basis, an outward recognition of quality performance freely given encourages growth of staff, and gradually new ideas are tested and tried. As often as the head nurse grows with encouragement and reinforcement, so must the role evolve. It must be defined and redefined again

and again, as the head nurse must be resocialized to her position.

4. Educational preparedness:
The value of educational preparation for head nurses in primary nursing cannot be underestimated. They must be knowledgeable about all primary nursing concepts in order to determine placement of patients and primary nurses. Head nurses must be as skilled as primary nurses in the five As and five Cs—authority, assertiveness, autonomy, accountability, advocacy, and continuity, commitment, communication, collaboration, coordination—for their decisions are the basis for planning and implementing quality health care. They also must be intuitive, a requirement not often found on job descriptions.

ASSESSMENT OF PATIENT NEED

Assessment of the nursing needs of patients is one of the first components to be determined in staffing for primary nursing. The measures that we have used consist of collecting data systematically and carefully on categories of patient care.[3]
Our classification system considers six areas of needs:
1. Patient care needs.
2. Observation.
3. Personal hygiene.
4. Therapeutics.
5. Reaction to illness and need for health teaching.

6. General medical/surgical back-up.

Levels of care are used in measuring areas of need: 1 indicates the lowest care level need, 4 indicates maximal care need.

It would be remiss to assume that this method of patient classification is complete. There are variables in patient care itself. The amount of physical and therapeutic care varies considerably from one seriously ill patient to another. Patients may be in minimal care categories and their needs for nonphysical professional care must be considered. Patients over 65 years of age require more nursing time than patients under 65.

Included among other variables in patient care are the patient census—its average and its variation—personal statistics, attributes of nursing care, definition of nursing practice, and the presence of supportive services such as service management.

Assessment of Nursing Needs

There are additional factors which must concern the head nurse in assessment of nursing needs of the patients:
1. Maintenance and promotion of health of the client.
2. Human adaptation and behavior.
3. Amount of contact the head nurse has with clients and families.
4. Coping mechanisms of the client.
5. Seasonal distribution of clients.

The dimensions of influence of these factors are far wider today be-

72 cause of advancement in the nursing profession.

Assessment of Nursing Resources

Carefully planned criteria and job descriptions are necessary to maintain optimal utilization of personnel and to conserve resources. The head nurse must also consider the following in her assessment of nursing resources, which will provide the basis of the

---

Carefully planned criteria and job descriptions are necessary to maintain optimal utilization of personnel and to conserve resources.

---

staffing system:

1. Level of involvement of nursing staff in other activities—day, evening or nights.
2. Weekend staffing—weekend activities and policies for weekends off.
3. Participation in committees and amount of inservice necessary.

DEVELOPING A STAFFING PATTERN

A staffing pattern, year-to-year, must be open and responsive to change. In developing a staffing pattern, the head nurse must take into account not only factors pertinent to traditional staffing patterns—is this patient ambulatory? Does he need a total bath? At what level of nursing care is he?—but the total manpower

TABLE 1
Primary Care Manpower Outline

Districts	7–3	3–11	11–7
I	Head Nurse, Primary Nurse, Associate Nurse	Charge Nurse, Associate Nurse	Charge Nurse, Associate Nurse
II	Primary Nurse, Associate Nurse	Associate Nurse	District Nurse
III	Primary Nurse, Associate Nurse, District Nurse	Associate Nurse	District Nurse
IV	Primary Nurse, Associate Nurse, Unit Aide*, Unit Clerk, Unit Clerk	Associate Nurse, Unit Aide**, Unit Clerk	Nurse's Aide
Capacity		40 Beds	
Average Occupancy		80%	
Average Census Daily		32	
Head Nurse	1	—	—
Charge Nurse	—	1	1
Primary Nurse	4	—	—
Associate Nurse	4	3	1
District Nurse	1	2	1
Nurse Aide	—	—	1
Unit Clerks	2	1	—
Unit Aides †	1	—	—
Nursing Care Coordinator †	0.5	—	—
Service Manager †	0.5	—	—

*½ Service Manager
**½ Nursing Care Coordinator
†5 day week or Supervisory

needed for delivery of primary care as well. Based on the number of districts, the head nurse must determine how

TABLE 2
Sample Budget Request Based on Manpower Need

Department Name	4 South	Department #	1978	Medical Surgical	
Position Title	Average Annual Salary per Position	Requested for each 24 hours	Requested FTE's (× 1.4)	Cost	Justification for Requests
Nrsg. Care Coord.*	14,000		.5	7,000	
Head Nurse	12,500	1	1.0	17,500	
Charge Nurse					
D	11,500		.4		
E	11,500	1	1.4	16,100	
N	11,500	1	1.4	16,100	
Primary Nurse	11,000	4	5.6	61,100	
Associate Nurse					
D	10,500	4	5.6	58,800	
E	10,500	4	5.6	58,800	
N	10,500	2	2.8	29,400	
District Nurse					
D	10,000		—		
E	10,000	1	1.4	14,000	
N	10,000	1	1.4	14,000	
Service Manager*	8,000		.5	4,000	
Unit Clerk					
D	6,000	2	2.8	16,800	
E	6,000	1	1.4	8,400	
N			—	—	
Unit Aide*					
D	5,500		1.0	5,500	
E	5,500		1.0	5,500	
Nurse Asst.					
N	5,500	1	1.4	7,700	
Total:			35.2		

#Beds 40 80% Capacity 32 daily—224 wkly.
*Requested for 5 day period only. Provides—5.0 Nsg. Hrs.

DIRECT NURSING FTEs
Days	9.0	Each date = 12.6 - 45%
Eves.	8.4	eve. = 8.4 - 30%
Nites	5.0	nite = 7.0 - 25%
Total	22.4	48 hr. = 28.0

many head, primary, associate, and district nurses are needed.

Table 1 outlines the manpower necessary to provide centralized primary care for patients on a 24-hour tour of duty on a routine medical/surgical nursing care unit with four districts. Table 2 is a sample budget request based on the manpower need determined in Table 1.

Some examples of justification of manpower needs that our head nurses and nursing care coordinators utilized this year were:

- Average census up from 26 patients to 32.
- Many isolation patients.
- Necessary to handle transfers.

Average daily census must also be considered in the determination of budget: is yearly census on a per annum basis 80 percent or 90 percent or 110 percent? It will often be necessary to acknowledge overall per annum bed capacity and then take 80 percent of those numbers and live within that budget.

Monitoring is necessary, not only on a yearly basis but daily. Figure 1 illustrates a routine nursing report used at Bayfront and completed every 24 hours. Note at the top of the report our determination of acuity of patient care. Primary nurses review the number of nursing hours required by their patients, determine whether the patients are classified 1, 2, 3, or 4, and head nurses identify the numbers and levels of staff on their unit. The bottom section of the report allows head nurses to include other pertinent factors which influence staffing, such as 12 patients going to surgery today or four patients in isolation. This daily control chart contains valuable information for our staffing clerk.

Staffing, above the range of normal, provides time to do extra things to strengthen the service. However, it is costly if such time occurs very frequently. Conversely, should it go the range of low normal with any consistency, remedial action of some kind must be found: for example, reducing the workload, streamlining procedures, or increasing staff.

At Bayfront Medical Center we use a daily, by-shift, staffing sheet which shows numbers and levels of nursing people on every unit and the census on every unit. The Daily Staffing Sheet identifies staffing needs to the staffing clerk on all three shifts. Specific information is requested:

1. What level of help is needed?
2. What are the expectations for the person requested?

All the information is recorded, and the entire staffing sheet and nursing service report are evaluated in order to properly reassign staff. Our monthly hours are also recorded from this sheet.

COMPARING DATA

The six-month national comparison by region by Hospital Administrative Services (HAS) of the American Hospital Association, affords a means of comparison for one's own data. Consultation service can accompany utilization of the HAS data if so desired. Caution must be used in such comparisons, however, as there must be the constant realization that nursing hours are far from standardized from hospital to hospital and there is a great range in how effectively nursing

There must be a constant realization that nursing hours are far from standardized from hospital to hospital and there is a great range in how effectively nursing time is conserved for purely nursing functions.

FIGURE 1. SAMPLE NURSING OFFICE REPORT

Unit_____
Date_____

	Classification					Staffing						
	1	2	3	4	Total	HN	CN	PN	AN	DN	NA	UA
7–3												
3–11	11											
11–7												

General Unit Information	7–3	3–11	11–7	Room	Acutely Ill and Deaths Name	Age	Diagnosis
Beginning Census							
Admitted							
Discharged							
Transferred Within							
Transferred In							
Transferred Out							
Deaths							
To OR							
From OR							
In Isolation							
Private Duty Nurses							
Ending Census							

Admissions—Transfers In

Time/Room	Patient	Age	Diagnosis	Doctor	Patient Condition

Unit Problems

76

time is conserved for purely nursing functions. In the case of timed procedures, this warning holds, because patient requirements should be based on clinical assessments of patients with particular clinical conditions, and on averages of a sufficient number of practices. All figures require periodic review.

SUPPORTING PRIMARY CARE PHILOSOPHY

Figure 2 illustrates a comparative example of productive nursing care hours at Bayfront Medical Center in 1974 and 1977.

Notice the differences in RNs and nursing assistants: In January 1974 the nursing assistant provided the majority—39 percent—of hands-on care. In 1977, eight percent of the care is rendered by nursing assistants.

The staffing pattern in 1974 allowed individuals to provide 3.7 nursing care hours per day. Our present centralized cyclical staffing patterns allow an average of 4.5 nursing care hours per day. According to Price, a complete cyclical staffing pattern includes:

1. Desired complement of personnel working each day.
2. Categories of personnel.
3. Shift work.
4. Days off.
5. Reduction in number and complement of personnel from work weekday to weekend that is appropriate for the needs of the specific unit.
6. Fair distribution of the desirable

and undesirable hours among all personnel.

7. A means of controlling utilization of the ever-increasing number of part-time employees for full and partial shift work.
8. Improved utilization of a float staff to enhance flexibility within the schedule and equalized staffing and fluctuation of patient needs and staff absences.[4]

In a comparison utilizing data collected at Bayfront Medical Center in 1974 and 1977, nursing care hours provided to patients on a routine medical/surgical unit indicate the primary system provides more nursing care hours:

Productive Hours

Functional 1974	Primary 1977
Nursing Care Hours (4-South)	Nursing Care Hours (4-South)
January 3.4	January 4.7
February 3.6	February 4.2
March 3.6	March 4.4

The numbers of nonprofessionals rendering service increased during 1976–1977. Managers say certain duties, such as emptying trash, water pitchers, ice pitchers, etc. are tasks more appropriately carried out by nursing assistants. Assigning these tasks to four nursing assistants allows the professionals to operate at the peak of their professional capacity.

There have been studies comparing cost effectiveness between team and primary systems. Marram has utilized comparisons of sick time and holiday, vacation and overtime hours.[5] Her

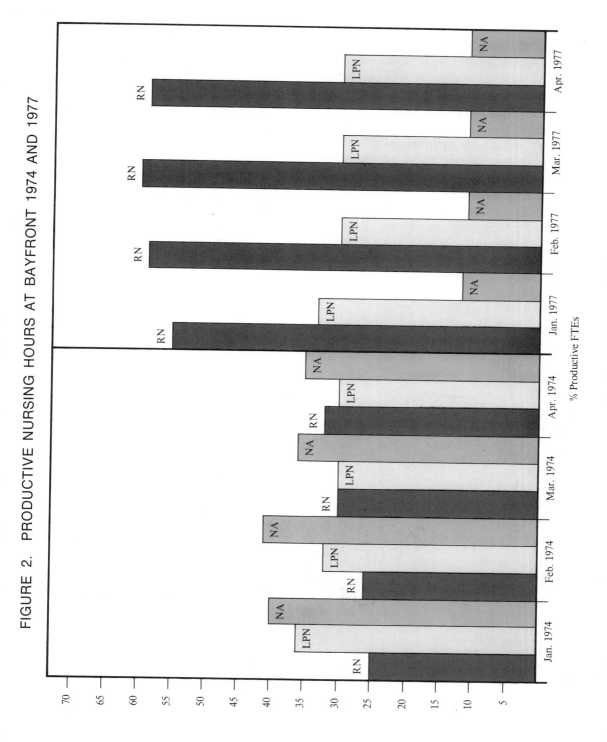

FIGURE 2. PRODUCTIVE NURSING HOURS AT BAYFRONT 1974 AND 1977

78

data reflect that the team unit cost the hospital more in time in everything but overtime hours. Primary nursing units consistently put in more overtime hours—87—but the team unit put in far more sick time. Our final projected staffing budget supports primary care philosophy:

- 58 percent care to be rendered by RNs.
- 32 percent care to be rendered by licensed practical nurses.
- 10 percent of care to be rendered by unit aides and nursing assistants.

In addition we have tried to encompass the following principles into our daily staffing practices:

"We believe that a hospital's greatest assets are its human assets, and the improvement of their value is both a matter of material advantage and moral obligation. We believe that employees must be treated as honorable individuals, justly rewarded, encouraged in their progress, fully informed, and properly assigned. Their lives and work must be given meaning and dignity, on and off the job."[6]

REFERENCES

1. *Accreditation Manual for Hospitals* (Chicago, Illinois: Joint Commission on Accreditation of Hospitals 1973) updated.
2. Ciske, K. "Primary Nursing: An Organization that Promotes Professional Practice." *Staffing: The Journal of Nursing Administration* (Wakefield, Mass.: 1974).
3. For elaboration on the establishment of primary care criteria, see NAQ 1:2 *Primary Nursing*.
4. Price, E. "Staffing for Patient Care." (New York: Springer Publishing Company, Inc. 1970) p. 102.
5. Marram, G. "The Comparative Cost of Operating a Team in Primary Nursing Care." *Journal of Nursing Administration* (May 1976).
6. Clarence, F. "Bits & Pieces." *The Economic Press* 10:4 (April 1977) p. 11.

Jane N. Fairbanks, R.N., M.S.
Senior Instructor
University of Colorado School of Nursing
Assistant Director of Nursing
University of Colorado Medical Center
  Hospital
Denver, Colorado

PRIMARY NURSING is the distribution of patient care so that the total care of an individual patient is the responsibility of one nurse, not many nurses. This concept proposes an arrangement of nurse and patient so that accountability can be identified and maintained for professional nursing practice. Although newly labeled "primary nursing," this arrangement is reminiscent of the case method of nursing assignments for patient care. In addition, it incorporates the strong components of responsibility and accountability into the role of the hospital nurse.[1] Because primary nursing is a vehicle that can allow nurses to work and develop at their highest professional level, it may prevent them from becoming discouraged and leaving the hospital for places in which they perceive they can practice as professional nurses.

The public is demanding health care services that are reflective of its personal needs. Primary nursing promotes individualized relevant patient care. The whole patient is the focus of the nurse and patients can and do perceive this personal care.

The decision was made to try primary nursing on a 30-bed acute general medical unit by the entire staff during a staff meeting in which goals for patient care were discussed. Nursing staff wanted more individual nursing care and consistent attention for the patients and their families and more job satisfaction for themselves. Once the nursing staff is committed to the concept of primary nursing care, it is the responsibility of the head nurse

80

Once the nursing staff is committed to the concept of primary nursing care, it is the responsibility of the head nurse to change the organization of the nursing unit to facilitate implementation of the concept.

to change the organization of the nursing unit to facilitate implementation of the concept.

Planning and staffing of a primary nursing unit, including scheduling, assignments, and arrangement of staff to work with primary patients are the foci of this article.

CHARACTERISTICS OF THE EXISTING UNIT

The unit in which this plan was implemented is within a 400-bed medical center hospital. Structurally, the unit is divided into two hallways with 15 patients in nine rooms on each side. Before implementation of primary nursing, staff switched assignments from one side of the hall to the other every few days with the exception of the team leaders who were permanently assigned to one side. Our analysis indicated that this arrangement made continuity of care very difficult.

The unit has 25 nursing service positions for patient care. This includes a head nurse, two team leaders, 12 registered nurses, two licensed practical nurses, and eight nursing assistants. The team leader position at this institution is unique. These two

nurses are appointed permanently to assist the head nurse in maintaining quality of patient care through administering patient care, observing staff functions, orientation of new staff members, and long-term planning for the unit. Before implementation of primary nursing, they also did much of the communication with other members of the health team, and had responsibility for most of the patient teaching and discharge planning. Several years ago, this unit chose to work the 4–40 work week, which means each staff member works four days per week, ten hours each day.

The Team Method

Prior to implementation of primary nursing, assignments were carried out according to the team nursing method. The permanent team leaders worked day shift doing most of the coordinating of patient care, visiting nurse referrals, and patient teaching. The evening and night shift each had two registered nurses who transcribed orders, administered medications, and completed other daily tasks. They were not accountable for any long-term care of patients. There were three auxillary staff during the day, two during the evening, and one during the night to assist with daily care. Although the basic scheduling could not change due to budget restraints, we determined that this system made poor use of the registered nurses' expertise and contained unreasonable expectations of the two team leaders.

Basic nursing tasks on the unit were accomplished; however, patients and families received sporadic attention. Teaching and emotional needs were considered according to the demands of the patient and/or the whims of the nursing staff. Therefore, some patients had many needs met and others had only immediate physical needs met. Although the team leaders attempted to do patient teaching, give the patient and family emotional support, and write nursing care plans, it was impossible for them to do this consistently for all 15 patients. Other staff nurses carried out some of the mentioned nursing care, but it was difficult to keep any one nurse accountable for any one task as each had a day off or was assigned to different patients.

STAFFING FOR PRIMARY NURSING

The following unit goals for patient care were identified at a staff meeting:
1. Interaction with every family.
2. Every patient treated as an individual.
3. Patient education.
4. Patient satisfaction.
5. Personal sense of satisfaction for nursing staff.

The unit staff and the head nurse examined these goals and decided that they were being achieved inconsistently and at varying levels. It was decided that implementation of primary nursing care was a feasible plan to accomplish these goals.

The primary nursing model described here is similar but not identical to Marram's.[2] Primary nurses work all three shifts. There are no associate nurses. Licensed practical nurses and nurse assistants are assigned to work with a registered nurse similar to Marram's "buddy" system. Each registered nurse-nurse assistant group is called a primary team. As LPNs become more comfortable with their abilities, they gain more independence and only consult with a registered nurse concerning their primary patients.

Preparing for Change

In preparation for the change to primary nursing, the unit began changing work patterns and nursing priorities. A major emphasis was placed on patient education. Inservices were presented to help staff arrange time for patient education in their busy day. Visiting nurse referrals were delegated by the team leader to other staff nurses. Ward clerks were prepared to order supplies and transcribe orders so staff nurses could give more time to patient care. Positive feedback was given by the head nurse to the staff for spending time with families and teaching patients,

Positive feedback was given by the head nurse to the staff for spending time with families and teaching patients, not just completing daily care and getting medications out on time.

82

not just completing daily care and getting medications out on time.

A task for the head nurse was to design the schedule with all staff assigned permanently to one side of the hall. Staff would then be able to administer care continuously to one group of patients. This was accomplished although there continued to be a few instances when someone had to switch sides due to illness, or other immediate staffing needs.

Appropriate use of our current registered nurses, licensed practical nurses, and nurse assistants was the next major decision to be made. The head nurse decided to arrange primary nurse teams of two. These two people, a registered nurse and a nurse assistant, work as a team, whether they are on one shift together or two different shifts. Registered nurses are held accountable for their primary patients' total nursing care and delegate to their team member as appropriate. Licensed practical nurses begin to work more independently with their patients as they are more comfortable. However, registered nurses always have final responsibility for their patients.

Each "primary team" has three "primary patients." The team is responsible for completing the nursing history, devising the plan of care, facilitating interaction with the family, coordinating with other members of the health team, offering emotional support, and planning for discharge of their primary patients.

The team leader no longer has responsibility for all 15 patients.

Registered nurses are responsible and accountable for their own patients.

Changing Responsibilities

Although we were not free to officially change the title of the team leader, we did change the responsibilities. They now function more as patient care coordinators and staff development people. They act as primary nurse role models, monitor staff to be sure appropriate care is done for the patient, and teach the staff nurses anything unfamiliar to them. They now facilitate rather than doing. The head nurse maintains quality patient care by conducting nursing rounds to make suggestions, monitoring written nursing care plans, and charting, providing consistent counseling and guidance of each staff member, and evaluating daily nursing care according to the goals for primary nursing.

Due to budget restraints, we were unable to increase the number of registered nurses per shift. Therefore, daily tasks continue to be carried out according to the total patient care concept. Staff members do as much as they can for the patients assigned to them; i.e., medications and treatments are done by the LPNs for the patients assigned to them.

Primary nurses continue to have responsibility for the total nursing plan of care. On a shift, nursing staff members are assigned to their own primary patients and the primary teams' plan of care on the others. For instance, if there is only one nurse assigned to one side of the hall, that nurse gives medications to all 15 patients. If other nurses are assigned to the same side of the hall, they give medications, do treatments, and administer physical care for their primary patients plus others assigned to them. The extra hour or so of time they have after completing daily tasks is spent with their primary patients teaching, counseling, etc., unless other patients have an immediate need. The other patients' long-term care is left for their primary nurses.

The staff decided that all shifts would have primary patients. Most people rotate to two shifts. This necessitates that the primary nurse who works nights delegates several tasks to the day nurse. Also, it should be noted that the night nurses choose patients whose care is more routine around the clock, such as comatose patients or those who tend to be awake for a period during the night for treatments.

Because the nurses work ten-hour days, all shifts have at least a two-hour overlap period. This allows for communication between primary nurse team members, such as registered nurses on the day shift and nurse assistants on the evening shift. It also allows for time for the night nurse to teach, or talk with physicians, since she is on the ward until 8:30 A.M. Afternoon overlap time is used for interaction with primary patients. The day nurse may monitor an intravenous infusion while the evening nurse teaches the primary patient.

Communication is a very important

Communication is a very important part of making this concept work. The use of the written nursing care plan in specific behavioral terms facilitates the primary nurses' plans being carried out by other shifts exactly as they planned.

part of making this concept work. The use of the written nursing care plan in specific behavioral terms facilitates the primary nurses' plans being carried out by other shifts exactly as they planned. Primary teams must find a way to communicate when they work different days. Many approaches seemed to be successful such as leaving notes and calling each other at home.

ADVANTAGES AND DISADVANTAGES

There are several advantages and disadvantages of this pattern for nursing care delivery.

Interaction with patients is significantly different on the unit as compared to pre-primary nursing days. Patients now get to know "their nurses" and wait for them "to return from a day off" to ask a question. One nurse is responsible for certain parts of the patient's care. Three or four nursing staff are not giving different directions to the family about dressing changes and four or five people are not talking with the patient about "his feelings about dying."

Morale and retention of nurse

84 assistants is a constant nursing administration problem. The primary nursing system allows a one-to-one relationship with a professional nurse for each nurse assistant, and therefore can increase learning, motivation, and satisfaction of the nurse assistant. A disadvantage for the nurse assistant is assignment to work with an unmotivated registered nurse or one who is uncomfortable with teaching and leadership.

The advantage for the registered nurse is that she can develop her leadership role on a one-to-one relationship with a nurse assistant rather than being thrust into a charge nurse-team leader position only to find that she does not have the basic skills to delegate, guide, teach, and facilitate patient care, as well as administer it. It quickly became evident that some registered nurses are not comfortable in their roles as teacher and leader. The head nurse was able to begin working immediately with these registered nurses on the specific problem areas observed.

Quality of care did improve. Patients know their medications and basic home care. Nursing care plans are completed more consistently. Families receive explanations and are included as a more significant part of the patients' care. Staff seem more satisfied, as Marram states.[3] It is hoped that retention will increase although it is too early to tell. Ciske states in one setting it did.[4]

A pre- and post-implementation study to evaluate patients' perceptions of how individualized their care is and nurses' satisfaction with their jobs is currently being conducted, but no data is available at this time.

Evaluation of Patients' Reactions

Evaluation of individual nursing staff has become much more objective and specific. Head nurses can evaluate the actual patient outcomes, observe the written care plan, and read the charting of each nurse's primary patients. They can also assess leadership potential and identify specific leadership weaknesses by observing registered nurses working with their team member.

Head nurses' ability to keep the staff accountable for each patient's care increased significantly. If a visiting nurse referral was not done or a patient not prepared for x-ray, the head nurses know exactly with whom to discuss the problem. They are also able to give specific positive feedback to staff based on observed patient outcomes.

Gwen Marram's study shows decreased cost on the primary nursing unit when comparing two units similar to the one currently under dis-

Evaluation of individual nursing staff has become much more objective and specific. Head nurses can evaluate the actual patient outcomes, observe the written care plan, and read the charting of each nurse's primary patients.

cussion.[5] This unit's cost remained the same as an identical medical unit practicing team nursing.

One general disadvantage can be that staff begin to say, "That's not my patient," or, "He is on the other side of the hall." We did not encounter this problem, but did spend significant time in staff meetings discussing the importance of team work. Another disadvantage is that any one staff member finds some patients particularly difficult to work with for long periods of time. This problem can be solved by changing primary nurses and explaining to the patients that the

new nurses have "new ideas to solve their problems."

Primary nursing is a system of patient care delivery arranged so that one professional nurse has responsibility and accountability for 24-hour care of a patient. Implementation of this system includes much planning on the part of nursing unit leaders. There are several administrative advantages of primary nursing which have been discussed. However, we must continue our diligent evaluation to be sure our quality care outcomes are positive, and that our utilization of staff is cost-effective.

REFERENCES

1. Manthey, Ciske, Roberton, and Harris "Primary Nursing." *Nursing Forum* IX: 1 (1970) p. 66.
2. Marram, G., Schlegel, M., and Bevis, E. *Primary Nursing* (St. Louis: The C. V. Mosby Co. 1974).
3. *Ibid.*
4. Ciske, K. L. "Primary Nursing, Evaluation."

American Journal of Nursing 74 (August 1974) p. 1437.
5. Marram, G. *Cost Effectiveness of Primary and Team Nursing*. (Wakefield, Mass.: Contemporary Publications 1976).

Standards + Nursing Care Needs = Staffing Methodology

Mary Naber, R.N., M.S.
Adminstrative Assistant

Janet Seizyk, R.N., M.S.
Associate Nursing Administrator
St. Joseph's Hospital
Milwaukee, Wisconsin

Nancy Wilde, R.N., B.S.N.
Assistant Director of Nursing
St. Michael Hospital
Milwaukee, Wisconsin

WITH PATIENT CARE becoming more and more complex, the responsibilities of nurses rapidly expanding and hospital costs constantly rising, we knew it was time to realistically evaluate the total workload in the nursing department and to take appropriate action to provide the needed patient care most effectively.

DESIGN, IMPLEMENTATION AND EVALUATION OF THE NURSING ACTIVITY MODEL

At St. Joseph's Hospital we believed that if existing standards could be made explicit in operational terms, and consistently applied, it would improve the ability of the hospital to provide appropriate staffing for needed nursing care hours and result in improved quality of nursing care, in the most economical way possible. We put our belief into action and, with a collaborative effort by systems development and nursing depart-

88

ments, a nursing activity study was initiated on ten medical/surgical units. The system which evolved was installed and evaluated on one test unit in March 1973, and subsequently implemented on the remaining nine units.

Defining Standards of Care

A committee composed of professional nurses was organized to define the standards of care to be applied in the determination of staffing. A table of nursing activities was developed by the committee. This table consisted of a listing of 571 activities performed by nursing personnel, and the estimated performance time and level of skill requirements per activity in accordance with a patient's classification.

Estimated "typical" performance time requirements were utilized—rather than time measurement—since we felt that measurement might reveal actual time spent yet fail to identify time required to do the task completely and well. Comparisons were made with the Commission for Administrative Services in Hospitals (CASH) study times, variances were discussed, and performance times of the activities adjusted if appropriate.[1] Performance time requirements were allocated for both predictable and nonpredictable activities based upon the typical time required to perform the identified activity.

Predictable activities were further broken down into those which were patient care category (PCC)-related and those which were not. The PCC-related activities were those documented on the patient's medication/treatment kardex, nursing care plan and/or team assignment record and scheduled for a particular time or shift. An average time for a patient in each of the four categories was arrived at by an analysis of those documents. Non-PCC-related activities (also referred to as unit activities) were those assigned activities not specifically related to a patient care category, such as narcotic count or shift report.

Nonpredictable activities were those unscheduled activities which were performed by nursing, such as answering a patient's call, prn dressing change, etc. Also included in this category was a personal, travel and delay factor.

Guidelines for Patient Care Criteria

Using Georgette's classification method as a major resource, the committee developed and tested guidelines to be utilized on each unit in the assessment and classification of each patient's condition and nursing care needs.[2] Nine areas of care, each given equal value, were designated: general health, eating, grooming, excretion, comfort, treatments, medications, teaching and emotional support. Specific action statements were required for the last two items and the needs of patient and/or family were to be considered. Four categories were used to identify total nursing needs utilizing the nine specified areas. The categories progressed from Category I: relative self-sufficiency, to Category IV: complete dependency.

Patients were categorized for the oncoming shift by RNs on the previous shift. The purpose for this was twofold: 1) to limit potential bias and 2) to provide an assessment of patient needs which would be available at the beginning of the shift.

Level-of-skill requirements were then based on the patients' overall category in accordance with the standards of care determined by the nursing committee.

With the completion of the activity table and the guidelines for patient care criteria, the project was well underway but nonetheless had a long, hilly and tortuous road ahead.

An Inhospital Study

Next came intense preparation for data collection: orientation of nursing personnel to the use of the guidelines to classify and report patient categories, initiation of an ongoing audit mechanism of classification to assure accuracy, development of input forms to handle data, preparation of written descriptions for conversion of data to computer programming, conduction of trial runs, recruitment and orientation of professional nurses to serve as on-unit observers, preparation of observer assignments and random observation schedules and the obtaining of needed supplies and equipment.

During the data collection phase, each of the ten medical/surgical nursing units was studied on all three shifts for seven consecutive days. Data collected included:

- Assignment information (derived

The old master staffing plan was based on a projected annual percentage of occupancy. As we all well know, census is only one determinant of staffing needs.

from the team assignment records, patients' nursing care plans and medication and treatment kardexes).
- Patient care category classification.
- On-unit observations (at randomly-selected intervals).
- Review of staffing as assigned versus staffing available.
- Review of patient turnover.

New Method of Staffing Determination

As had been anticipated through the data base collected, a new method of staffing determination was born, to be readied for installation and evaluation. The old master staffing plan was based on a projected annual percentage of occupancy. As we well know, census is only one determinant of staffing needs.

A critical factor uncovered in our study was that the performance time requirements for a specific patient category was unique for each of the ten nursing units. This provided validation for that "gut feeling" (called nursing intuition by some) that staffing requirements differed significantly for the various departmental service patients (for example, medical versus surgical or orthopedics).

The revised master, monthly and daily staffing plans for each unit were based on the described historical data of each unit's six-month profile of patient category mix, with performance time and level-of-skill requirements related to the specific patient category as well as to the percentage of occupancy.

Approval was given by administration to install the system, renamed the nursing activity model, on a unit where overall staffing was to be decreased on 7 to 3:30 and 3 to 11:30 shifts and increased on 11 to 7 shifts— the result being an overall staff reduction.

Staff conferences and staff development sessions were conducted immediately before and throughout the three-month test installation period. The major impact, other than staffing, was the change required in assignment of patient care, using the table of nursing activities as a guide to assure the assignment of personnel according to the patient's classification and needs, rather than according to the "tasks to be performed."

Benefits

To evaluate the effectiveness of the system, data was collected and analyzed in the same manner as in the original study (but on one unit rather than ten) and compared with the original study findings. Additional criteria used to evaluate the installed system's effect on patient care included a before and after installation review of incident reports, study of omitted activities, the nursing audit, a correlated patient/personnel questionnaire survey and a daily staffing report which compared staffing available against the shift's staffing requirements in accordance with that shift's patient category mix.

We were elated with the benefits achieved as identified after installation:

- Overall decrease (four percent) on all shifts, in nonproductive hours.
- Decrease (43 percent) in incident reports.
- Improved nursing care plans (quality and currency).
- Increase in quantity and quality of nursing rounds, especially 11–7 shift.
- Initiation of group patient preoperative teaching.
- Improved assignment of personnel in accordance with level-of-skill requirements.
- Decreased omission of assigned activities.
- Decreased RN absenteeism.
- Increased staff development in accordance with needs.
- Additional job satisfaction reported by some personnel.
- Problem solving at the unit level.
- Cost reduction.
- Nursing audit reports revealed: Improved performance in assignment, teaching and RN admission notes.
- Patient/personnel questionnaires revealed no significant overall change by patients or personnel on either the "control unit" or the test unit. Both before and after implementation, patients on each

unit viewed the care as adequate and also more positively than did personnel, even though the staff on the test unit was reduced. (The questionnaire dealt with the provision of a healthful climate, direct ministrations and communications, protection of patients' rights and administrative aspects.)

Though the patients on the test unit did not perceive a change in care, personnel responses reflected RNs' increased involvement in personnel assignments, planning patient care, patient teaching and planning for patient discharge (continuity of care).

Problems?

Yes, there were problems; however, not all the problems encountered were due to the system. The system brought many problems to the surface, into clearer focus, and brought about meaningful action to at least initiate resolution. Among those problems identified were:

- Inability to meet peak loads with appropriate level of skill.
- Lack of RN understanding and/or acceptance of their professional roles. (Some preferred the "medication nurse" role and were reluctant to delegate the task where appropriate to the LPN or RN assigned to care for the patient. In other situations, RNs assigned nonprofessional personnel to patients who should have been assigned to RNs. Desk tending was difficult for some to release. Additionally, the need for

RNs to assess, plan, provide and evaluate patient needs and patient care, and to provide staff development for the non-professional staff, was not always viewed as within their job scope.)
- Lack of LPN/Nursing Assistants' understanding and/or acceptance of their roles (by law and nursing standards set).

(Personnel were viewing the *task only* as criteria for assignment rather than the condition of the patient for whom the task was to be performed. Previously, due to lack of available appropriate staff, the non-professional personnel had been overutilized and, with proper staff available, were being assigned more appropriately in accordance with their skill and training and according to patient needs.)
- Inaccurate reporting of staff hours available.
- Inadequate communication between shifts and part-time workers.
- Reduced job satisfaction felt by some LPNs and Nursing Assistants (due to loss of job content).
- Continued resistance to change.

In the eyes of those of us responsible for its "early days," the system, though still requiring some growing up and maturing, was ready to seek new guardianship and reach for new horizons. The amber light changed to green, and hospital administration gave approval for the system to be

92 fully implemented on the remaining nine units studied. This was accomplished with relative ease. Responsibility for maintenance was transferred from the systems development department to the nursing department.

MAINTENANCE OF THE NURSING ACTIVITY MODEL

Utilizing a staffing methodology which includes complexity of care as well as census, which is dependent on a patient care classification completed by the RN caring for the patient and which strives for quality by matching the knowledge and skill of the practitioner with the needs of the patient, makes one feel very fortunate. There is a satisfaction in having the capability to graphically display complexity of care trends next to census to justify staffing increases or decreases. The application of a standard guideline for patient care classification has achieved a consistent measurement of complexity. Previous assessment of care needs was variable dependent on each RN's level of knowledge and experience. Articulating staffing requirements for administrative approval is a more logical and objective process with the rationale for requests based on patient needs and data accu-

In an era of cost consciousness, nursing personnel, who comprise a large segment of the budget, need to be viewed in terms of possible cost containment and certainly cost effectiveness.

mulated for each nursing unit per shift and day of the week.

In an era of cost consciousness, nursing personnel, who comprise a large segment of the budget, need to be viewed in terms of possible cost containment and certainly cost effectiveness. Is the right person caring for the right patient? Assignments can be analyzed if they include category of patient as well as worker. A typical preemployment question is: "What is the usual number of patients per assignment?" The answer is dependent on numbers and categories of patients.

Personnel Orientation

Maintenance activities are essential to the credibility of the staffing methodology. These activities fall into the general categories of personnel orientation, audits and updating of documents. All personnel require orientation to the objectives of patient classification as it affects staffing and patient care assignments. The RNs particularly need to know end results of classification and the importance of current patient care plans and medication/treatment kardexes which are source documents for classification. All RNs are oriented to the patient care classification procedure.

Updating the Master Staffing Pattern

Head nurses perform periodic assignment and classification audits enabling them to identify staff nurses requiring assistance and conveying to their staff the importance of accurately completing the procedure. In conjunction with budget preparation, head nurses annually update the master staffing patterns using the most recent six-month unit profile. Nursing supervisors audit patient care categories and assignments twice per month on each shift for every nursing unit. The audit reports are forwarded to nursing administration for analysis of problem areas. Erroneous staffing requirements are derived from a high error rate. If the error rate persists, the unit profile (the base for master staffing) is inaccurate. The goal is to classify every patient on each shift, creating a large data base that is not dramatically influenced by occasional errors. The daily staffing requirements form is used on each shift by supervisors for float staff assignment and to reassign staff from units of lesser to greater need.

Documents that require maintenance are: table of nursing activities, performance time requirement table, unit profile and patient care category guidelines. The table of nursing activities can be updated retrospectively through committee or concurrently through reports from procedure and policy committee chairmen. A review of patient care plans and medication/treatment kardexes, with extraction of nursing activities for each category of patient, determines the currency of the performance time requirement table. A sampling of each category of patient per shift and unit is taken. The unit profile is updated at the beginning of each fiscal year to correspond with data used to develop master staffing for that particular fiscal year. Since the data for all documents is on computer file, all changes are forwarded to data processing using forms and procedures developed by them. The guidelines of patient care criteria are reviewed and revised as necessary.

MODIFICATION AND ADAPTATION OF THE NURSING ACTIVITY MODEL IN ANOTHER HOSPITAL SETTING

St. Joseph's Hospital and St. Michael Hospital not only have the same sponsoring body—the Franciscan Sisters of Wheaton, Illinois—but are also served by a single board of directors. Sharing of services between the two institutions has long been encouraged, thus it was natural for the two hospitals to work together in the expansion of the system to St. Michael's.

A project committee composed of RNs was formed and the St. Michael Hospital project instructor, well-oriented as to the methodology and mechanics of the system, guided the committee in the preliminary modifications necessary in the table of nursing activities and guidelines for patient care criteria to adequately reflect the hospital's nursing philosophy and standards of practice. Minimal modification of the already developed computer programming was necessary to effectively process the data to be collected.

The nursing activity model has been adapted to the specialty areas—critical care, obstetrics and pediatrics—with some minor modifications in the guidelines for patient care criteria.

94 With the "discovery" of the need for a well-documented nursing care plan to identify patient needs, the format and content requirements of the nursing kardex was redesigned for use on all nursing units. Assignment sheets were also standardized throughout the nursing department.

Guidelines for Psychiatric Patients

Arriving at realistic patient performance time for the psychiatric area was somewhat more complicated. A unique set of guidelines had to be developed and tested in order to adequately assess the levels of dependency of these patients. The final product consists of only seven areas of care, since eating, grooming and excretion were combined under one heading, "Basic Physical Needs." The revised guidelines, while recognizing physical needs of the patient, place emphasis on the psychosocial component of care.

A table of 62 psychiatric nursing activities was developed giving specific attention to nursing actions and corresponding performance time required for specific patient behaviors. The frequency with which these activities would be carried out is documented on the nursing care plan as are other nursing interventions.

Staffing Requirements

A further modification was needed and accomplished in integrating the system with primary nursing concepts. This required level-of-skill designations in accordance with the standards of care set for primary nursing.

A simplified daily staffing requirements report has been incorporated into the "24-hour nursing service report," so that pertinent information is included on one computerized report sheet (rather than two). This provides nursing administration with a comprehensive overview of the specific unit's staffing needs (either excess or deficit) in relationship to the patient's condition on a more timely basis. It reinforces to the staff that the classifications are being utilized and facilitates necessary staffing adjustments prior to start of the next shift.

Maintenance Requirements

Maintenance requirements, as described previously, are substantially the same with our modified system but the critical monitoring of patient classification perhaps bears reiteration. The head nurses are held responsible for the audit, and weekly reports are submitted to nursing service. This reinforces the role of head nurses as first-line supervisors and, since they have a responsibility for determining staffing needs, they must have input into and knowledge and control over the factors that influence these needs.

Problems

Our experience thus far has been that variations in staffing needs occur more often due to staff illness or vacation than as a result of a change in patient mix. However, if a significant change in patient mix were to

Our experience thus far has been that variations in staffing needs occur more often due to staff illness or vacation than as a result of a change in patient mix.

develop, the data would be available to make the appropriate needed change in staffing.

Until a hospital-wide commitment was made, and because results and gratification were not immediate, frustration, anxiety and hostility had to be worked through in the early stages of implementation. Responsibility for the project resting in the nursing department was helpful in gaining acceptance and support. Intensity and volume of nursing in-service needed was understandably high. Additionally, the orientation of other departments and persons, including medical staff, must be considered prior to implementation of a system which impacts patient care through so many disciplines.

Benefits

The nursing activity model has proved invaluable to us as a tool in justifying budgetary staffing requests. It has made quality nursing care more than just a potential. It has also served us well in communications between the nursing office and the staff on a nursing unit when reassignment of personnel is necessary to or from a unit. The decision becomes more acceptable when the rationale is known and understood.

The benefits achieved have made it all worthwhile. Twelve inpatient units are now on the system, and their master staffing budgets for 1977–1978 have been determined by the statistics generated by the nursing activity model.

EVALUATION FOR THE FUTURE

The involvement and commitment of a wide spectrum of professional staff in the development, implementation, evaluation and monitoring of the system had a direct correlation to its success. But beyond the usual "acceptance" factor, it has yielded totally unexpected benefits. In retrospect, there is evidence of a gradual increased awareness and clarification of the head nurse role and improvement in job performance. Head nurses and clinical coordinators (supervisors) were vital components in determining success or failure of all aspects of the system. They actively participated in the interpretation and support of the system to members of the staffs. By necessity, they became involved in determination and interpretation of standards, evaluation of care plans, patient classifications and assignment of personnel. They served as a stimulus to developing improved communication between shifts and all categories of workers. They also became more aware of the staff development needs of personnel and assisted in determining how to best provide the needed training. All of these factors resulted in their own staff development, greater understanding

96

This nursing activity model is now recognized as a highly effective tool which serves as a guideline to effective staffing and a sensitive indicator of the impact of changing conditions on hospital costs.

of their roles and effectiveness in job performance.

The system is highly dependent upon quality assessment of patient needs, communication of the plan to meet these needs in terms of a well-developed nursing care plan and reliability of patient classification. If these conditions are met, the utilization of the methodology described provides factual translation of patient needs and delivery into credible staffing guidelines. The availability of appropriate staff, proper assignment and ongoing monitoring are then necessary to provide the required patient care identified.

This nursing activity model is now recognized as a highly-effective tool which serves as a guideline to effective staffing and a sensitive indicator of the impact of changing conditions on hospital costs. It has facilitated and enhanced communication between nursing and hospital administration.

A Potential Billing System

The potential exists for initiating charges for nursing services based on patient care categories. A billing system that initiates a separate charge for nursing services would provide nursing with the opportunity of ap-

pearing on the revenue side of the ledger instead of only expense and would make visible nursing's contribution to health care. It would also be an equitable way of charging patients for nursing services received rather than for room accommodation.

Future Revisions

The overall system in its present form meets the requirements originally set for it, is adaptable to all in-patient nursing service areas and is highly cost effective; however, it is somewhat cumbersome and requires a highly skilled person for data collection and interpretation. In its current state, knowledge of the intricacies of the system and the computer programs, through which the data is processed, is critical to valid output. The model has been revised conceptually within the systems development department collaboratively with financial administration and the two nursing departments. The revised model will continue to use the nursing care plan and unit profile as the major source documents. Additionally, revision will include:

- Elimination of observations, the most costly and difficult aspect in terms of human resources. (Nonpredictable performance time factor, derived from observations, accounted for only approximately 15 percent of the total staffing requirements. An "automatic" 15 percent nonpredictable factor will be included.)
- Converting maximum amount of manual processing to automation.

- Planning for on-line computer processing of data.
- Provision for the ability to study any or all of the staffing factors, a single unit or shift with a minimum of manpower effort and time lag from point of request to reported results.

A planned audit mechanism to assure quality care plans, accurate patient classification, assignment of personnel, maintenance of an updated table of nursing activities and monitoring of the unit profile reports will be critical to the success of the ongoing maintenance of the system.

97

REFERENCES

1. Commission for Administrative Services in Hospitals. "A Study of Nursing Time Requirements for Patients of Various Age Groups" (California: 1966) Unpublished.

2. Georgette, J. "Staffing by Patient Classification." *Nursing Clinics of North America* (Philadelphia: W. B. Saunders Co. June 1970).

SUGGESTED READINGS

Aydelotte, M. K. *Nurse Staffing Methodology* (Washington, D.C.: U.S. Department of Health, Education and Welfare, Publication No. (NIH) 73–433. 1973).

Bihldorff, J. P., McPhail, A., Payne R. and Scanlon, R. "An Approach to Patient Classification . . . and Some Results." *Hospital Administration in Canada* (February 1976) p. 22–25.

Christie, L. S., S.R.N., R.M.N. "Researching Staffing Needs in Psychiatric Hospitals." *Nursing Times* (November 28, 1974) p. 1870–71.

Stevens, B. J. "What is the Executive's Role in Budgeting for Her Department?" *Hospitals* (November 16, 1976) p. 83–86.

On the Scene:
A Family-Centered Approach to Staffing

DEVELOPING A COMPREHENSIVE NURSING CARE SYSTEM

Organization and staffing of nursing services at Family Hospital has changed in an orderly and deliberately controlled fashion from a hierarchical traditional system of multiple levels to one of decentralized autonomy and accountability for individual clinical specialization. To date, the change process is incomplete. However, the process has been intended to eliminate the role and title of head nurse and supervisor as the family care system is refined to provide direct clinical responsibility and accountability by each professional nurse for a given patient and family.

Changing the Administrative Role

The role change began three years ago with the hiring of the first clinical specialist, who had the difficult task of overcoming the traditional nursing supervisory role image. Today, each clinical service has a clinical expert nurse responsible for the quality of care provided by the nursing staff. Some clinical directors are prepared on a graduate level in their specialty area, while others are clinical experts through their experience in advanced clinical preparation.

To fill the administrative role, knowledge and application of the art and science of administration is required. At Family Hospital, every nurse is provided the opportunity to grow and develop in this area of accountability and responsibility.

In order to create this change fully utilizing RNs in the direct care-giving system of family-centered care, significant numbers of nurses had to be added to the staffing pattern at Family Hospital. This change required significantly new programs in recruitment.[1]

As the need for RNs increased, the change from a care-giving system, which utilized nursing assistants and team methodology, to one in which there is full implementation of primary nursing, required a new approach to staffing. This approach involved hiring an individual oriented to personnel management and

---

To fill the administrative role, knowledge and application of the art and science of administration is required. At Family Hospital, every nurse is provided the opportunity to grow and develop in this area of accountability and responsibility.

---

guidance and counseling of other individuals, rather than an RN.

In our family-centered care approach, the job of the RN changes considerably, from administration to direct patient care. Each patient and family is assigned a family care nurse, an RN who maintains coordination of care for the duration of the hospital stay. This means that each patient is assured of having an RN responsible for planning, *giving* and evaluating his own care.

Changing Recruitment Goals

Four years of work and effort went into changing our nursing service. As I review those years in an attempt to share with a reader audience the methodologies that were employed, I realize it is quite difficult to share the totality of the change. It is clear that change has taken place. In 1973, there were 62 permanent full time or part time RNs, 120 nursing assistants and 35 licensed practical nurses for this 220-bed acute care hospital. There were obvious violations of state nursing care standards, including the delegation of RN functions to LPNs. Many of the staff had been hired with no commitment to work evenings, nights or weekends. Temporary agency nurses were employed regularly in such key positions as night supervision. The dilemma confronting me was how could we possibly attract nurses to this environment? In order to change direction, we had to find nurses who would accept responsibility and accountability for patient care 24 hours a day, 7 days a week.

The nurse recruitment goals were not difficult to define. Attaining them was another matter. The joint effort of nurse recruiters and the personnel department is a key factor toward our ability to attract RNs.

The nurse recruitment goals were not difficult to define. Attaining them was another matter. The joint effort of nurse recruiters and the personnel department is a key factor toward our ability to attract RNs.

Changing Other Roles

Changes in leadership roles, changes in staff nurse roles and strengthening a total organization for the delivery of nursing services were required to lay the foundation for effective staffing. In that strengthening, a new nursing leader—Joanne D. Wall—was brought into the organization in 1975 as the Director of Nursing. As Assistant Administrator for Patient Care Services for Family Hospital and Nursing Home, there are two nursing directors and ten department heads in addition to nursing reporting to me. These additional departments relate to the direct patient care services, such as physical, occupational, speech and recreation therapy, among others.

Today, Family Hospital's nursing service consists of 139 RNs called family care nurses; 19 RNs as clinical directors and in other supportive administrative positions; 14 LPNs; 55 family care assistants and 16 ward clerks.

Our turnover rate has decreased significantly. Nursing personnel are leaving for reasons other than job dissatisfaction, such as relocation, pregnancy, etc.

Orderly Transition

Transition has been orderly. No individual in any position was terminated in order to make room for others. Many of the nursing staff have preceded me in their tenure at Family and persevered through organizational change that helped to evolutionalize our health care system. Indebtedness to their continuous work efforts and support in maintaining a stable environment through change is continuously expressed.

While we have not achieved a perfect marriage between the needs of patients and staff, we have come a long way in bringing them together. In order to develop a concept of staffing which is sensitive to patients and staff, serious thought was given to what system of staffing or combination of systems could be utilized. A number of concepts have been discarded, some incorporated, and some are presently being combined. Effective yet sensitive staffing is a process that is never completed but constantly developing.

We, as the staff at Family, recognize that we have grown in developing a comprehensive nursing care system that has been a lifelong ideal for many nurses. We recognize that we still have many improvements to make in our family-centered care system and hope that other nurses in other hos-

102 pitals will be working with us toward accomplishment of better nursing care through staffing and improved utilization of RNs in a direct care-giving setting.

REFERENCE

1. Brown, B. "How to Succeed in Recruiting." *American Journal of Nursing* 76:4 (April 1976).

Barbara Brown, R.N., Ed.D., F.A.A.N.
Patient Care Services Administrator
Family Hospital
Milwaukee, Wisconsin

STAFFING: AN ADMINISTRATIVE PERSPECTIVE

The single most significant ingredient in the health care enterprise is its human resources. Essential to successful provision of nursing care is the creative and relevant utilization of nursing staff. A nursing service department often accounts for over 60 percent of the hospital staff and over 50 percent of the hospital's salary allocations. Family Hospital is no exception.

The staffing activity, therefore, is one which is crucial. It involves sound planning in order to correlate the available personnel with the consumer needs and resulting services offered to patients and families in an acute care setting.

Cost Effective Delivery

At the foundation of our approach to cost effective delivery of nursing care are several beliefs:

1. The family-centered care philosophy is a constant in refining the nature and modes of nursing care.
2. For continued cost effective care those proximal to care delivery must be involved in the design, implementation and evaluation of staffing patterns and related regulations.
3. Consumer evaluation of our patient care is essential for it to continue to be responsive to the needs of our patient populations.

In evolving a family-centered care approach which reflects consultative

We have experienced an opportunity to combine the centralized and decentralized systems of staffing. RNs who comprise three-fourths of the nursing staff assume responsibility for sustaining mutually agreed on budget allocations.

sensitive care, and is representative of exemplary assessment and intervention, the number of professional nursing staff has been increased while the number of nonprofessional supportive nursing staff has been decreased. We have experienced an opportunity to combine the centralized and decentralized systems of staffing. RNs who comprise three-fourths of the nursing staff assume responsibility for sustaining mutually agreed on budget allocations. Staff nurses are supported in this activity with direction from their immediate supervisors (clinical directors) and the consultation and coordination effort of an administrative assistant for staffing. Our administrative assistant is uniquely qualified with a social work and systems management background. By reducing management layers, and thus decreasing cost generated by numbers of supervisory personnel, dollars can be reinvested at the care giver level.

Patient Care Hour Allocation

In this setting we use a patient care hour allocation which relates the hours of care per day needed by a prescribed patient population to the number of patients present. All participate in design of flexible staffing patterns which best tap the talents of professional staff including the immediate supervisor as a care giver.

A focus only on position control, while it places numbers of people in a clinical area, does not take into account such variables as:

- Changing census (a reality in most hospitals).
- Length of stay and therefore frequency of admissions and discharges which significantly affects specific nursing activities.
- Method of assignment, that is, caseload vs. functional or team assignments.
- Classification of patient and family needs significantly affecting the quantity and nature of nursing care provided.
- Geographical design and size of nursing units.
- Availability of support services

within and external to the nursing service department.

Therefore, the patient care hour figure assists in determining needed manhours based on average census and for computing "guide" numbers of positions for yearly budgeting activities.

Nursing service departments, in seeking their directions for the future, have an obligation to clearly define patient care programs based on changing needs of patient and family populations. They must collaborate with other disciplines with the hospital and involve staff at all levels in designing use of resources. Further, nursing service departments must provide environments in which professional nursing practice can grow and where individual nursing staff can make a meaningful contribution compatible with their own beliefs and capabilities.

Joanne D. Wall, B.S.N., M.S.
Director of Nursing Service
Family Hospital

STAFFING PATTERNS

Twenty-four hour professional staffing in hospitals is a fact of life for nurses. Ideal working hours, such as nine to five, Monday through Friday with weekends off, are impossible unless all patients could be sent home on off-hours.

In order to attract and maintain

103

104   highly-skilled nurses, hospitals must remain flexible in staffing and be willing to consider the needs of nurses as people. Unless nurses are used within their capabilities, their energies will be diverted, influencing their effectiveness.

The frustration of inadequate staffing can be avoided. Family Hospital recognizes that all units cannot operate under the same pattern because of the diversity of patient and personnel needs within each unit. To understand how Family Hospital differs in their staffing patterns, it is necessary to take a brief look at staffing methods.

Staffing must take into consideration the training and competence of the nursing personnel and the types of patient needing care. For example, in the labor and delivery area nurses must have the clinical expertise to assist the mother in the childbirth experience. If there is more than one mother delivering at a given time, it is necessary to have an adequate number of nurses available to provide the required care.

Additional nursing staff will be needed after the deliveries to provide care for the new infants. Special problems of the mother and infant will also make a difference in the number and type of staff needed. Acuity of illness, diagnosis, age and number of treatments will affect all patient care required and the number of staff necessary to supply that care.

How do most hospitals handle these problems? Current methods involve centralized or decentralized staffing.

Centralized Staffing

Centralized staffing assigns one person in the nursing administration office to plan coverage for all nursing units. A master staffing pattern is developed for these units and staffing is based on a pre-established standard. This staffing coordinator has access to clerical help to type, process and distribute the master plan to the units. The coordinator knows the number and availability of staff on any given day and therefore is able to make the necessary day-to-day changes when sickness or other emergencies occur. The coordinator is able to do this by rotating nurses from one floor to another to achieve the best coverage throughout the hospital. Such a person is important in keeping nurses involved in nursing rather than nonnursing functions.

The pitfalls of centralized staffing patterns are many. The staffing coordinator unaware of the implications of clinical problems, may not understand that nurses need certain clinical expertise if they are rotated to more specialized units. Nurses are often placed into regimented schedules, offered no choices and few options for change. They are not included as part of the decision-making process, which leads them to frustration and feelings of helplessness and insignificance.

Decentralized Staffing

Decentralized staffing has helped to solve some of these frustrations. Nurses have more input into staffing patterns because the responsibility for staffing is entrusted to the unit supervisor, who is aware of the clinical needs and the personal needs of the staff nurses. However, because the supervisor is not an expert in staffing methods and does not have access to clerical help, long tedious hours are spent in nonnursing functions. The schedule remains confusing and inconsistent in spite of sincere efforts.

Family Hospital has attempted to solve the frustrations of staffing by combining the advantages of centralized and decentralized methods. In order to do this, the position of administrative assistant for staffing has evolved. This position is more a consultative and personnel/managerial role rather than a functional or task-oriented role. Each unit is given the option of using this person as a valuable resource in developing their own staffing pattern. As a result, several staffing patterns have taken shape at Family Hospital.

Self Staffing

One of these staffing patterns has developed in the New Life Center. The clinical director was faced with a large number of part time staff, inadequate coverage of P.M.s and nights,

---

Self staffing allows the nurses on the unit to assign themselves on the work schedule while assuming total responsibility for daily coverage of the unit and maintenance of the appropriate level of competency.

---

three permanent day people who did not rotate to other shifts, and diversity in competence and expertise. It was felt that a structured staffing pattern could not meet the clinical needs *and* the personal needs of the staff. The problem was presented to the staff and they agreed to assume the responsibility for self staffing.

Self staffing allows the nurses on the unit to assign themselves on the work schedule while assuming total responsibility for daily coverage of the unit and maintenance of the appropriate level of competency. Self staffing involves group cooperation, sensitivity to peer needs, individual accountability and an awareness of the coverage needed in a 24-hour period. Self staffing takes advantage of the best of centralized staffing and decentralized staffing. With this combined system, clerical work and day-to-day problems can be handled by the administrative assistant for staffing with direct input from the unit.

GUIDELINES

The following guidelines were set up to make self staffing work effectively. In a group meeting, the nurses on a unit decide how many nurses are needed to give safe care to their patients. The nurses then identify: full time and part time nurses; nurses working permanent P.M.s and nights; nurses who will work days with rotations to P.M.'s and/or nights; and nurses working eight-hour or ten-hour shifts.

Given the number of rotations that

106

must be made to P.M. and night shifts, the nurses fill in these rotations prior to filling in day hours. This is important since P.M. and night coverage is the hardest to fill. Rotations are done in blocks of three days to develop some consistency and flow from days to P.M.s or nights.

Permanent full time and part time nurses fill in their hours making sure their staffing pattern includes every other weekend. Part time nurses working less than 20 hours a week must work one weekend a month. They should try working the weekend where coverage is most needed.

The schedule is usually made out five to six weeks in advance at a group meeting to allow for adequate planning time for staff.

ADVANTAGES AND DISADVANTAGES

Advantages of self-staffing cited by the staff are that it enables them to arrange their personal lives more conveniently; allows flexibility for "moms" who need days off when children are out of school for teachers conferences; allows for dental and doctor appointments on a more predictable basis; and allows for a choice to work with other nurses they are more compatible with.

Disadvantages cited were that nurses filling in the schedule last are not always given first chance on succeeding schedules; there is inadequate coverage or too much coverage on the same days with staff unwillingness to "give and take"; there is not always available staffing to meet the needs of the unit; and the last person to fill in

The clinical director of one of the units sees herself as a consultant in identifying the limitations or problems the group does not identify. She facilitates decision making by clarifying the problem and defining alternative solutions.

the schedule sometimes has less flexibility unless this can be discussed with other staff members.

CHOOSING ALTERNATIVES

An interview with the clinical director of one of the units utilizing self staffing gives us insight into her role. She sees herself as a consultant in identifying the limitations or problems the group does not identify. She facilitates decision making by clarifying the problem and defining alternative solutions. For example, a nurse working ten-hour shifts four days a week wanted to work two days, have two days off, work two days, have one day off. This preference did not work well for continuity of patient care. The alternatives were stated. Work all four days in a row and have three days off or work every other day. The first alternative was chosen.

The clinical director also calls emergency meetings of the unit as a group to solve crises. For example, on a 35-bed medical service the patient census rose rapidly in January 1977. It was decided that two night nurses were necessary to give safe patient care. The *group* decided how they would rotate to cover this crisis situation. On the New Life Center unit, three nurses were necessary to cover nights. One nurse decided she could not handle frequent rotations from days to P.M.s and nights so she volunteered to go to full time nights, if she could have every Thursday and Friday night off. The group agreed to cover every Thursday and Friday night.

There are pitfalls that can deveop in self staffing. Failure can be imminent if staff members are immature, do not have a sense of caring for their fellow workers, the ability to compromise, a commitment to their patients and their nursing responsibilities, or if they do not attend the unit meetings.

However, the advantages of a flexible staffing pattern far outweigh the disadvantages in our experience at Family Hospital. Nurses using the group process and staffing guidelines can nurture and enhance the sense of caring and bonding between each other. The group process allows for identification of preferences, discussion of individual needs and compromise to provide solutions to staffing needs. The staff quickly sees results directly related to their efforts, which enhances their feelings of significance and decreases their feelings of helplessness or lack of control.

Individual freedom of choice is one of the oldest human rights but has assumed less and less importance as the nurses have become more institutionally oriented. Institutional goals have taken precedence over individual needs. We feel that at Family Hospital self staffing has been a good begin-

ning in promoting freedom of choice, higher motivation and professional satisfaction.

Barbara Van Offeren, R.N., M.S.N.
Clinical Director

Carol Glynn, R.N., M.S.N.
Clinical Director
New Life Center
Family Hospital

THE ROLE OF THE STAFFING OFFICE AT FAMILY HOSPITAL

Centralized or decentralized staffing—these are the two choices that have been open to nursing service administrators. Decentralized staffing has been criticized as an improper utilization of the professional nurses' time. Centralized staffing was considered the answer to the concern of improper utilization of nurses. However, when the responsibility for hours is removed from the unit, individual sense of responsibility for adequate staffing is also removed.

From Centralized to Decentralized Staffing

As did many hospitals, Family Hospital decided to implement centralized staffing. All schedules were made out through the nursing service office. The staff used a system of forms to indicate any special requests they might have. Any problems with staffing—such as call-ins, needs due to vacant positions and adjustments to daily staffing—were handled by staffing's administrative assistant.

107

108 In August 1974, staffing regulations were developed by an ad hoc committee after meeting with staff from all levels and all shifts. The regulations included expectations for weekend, holiday shift and floor rotation, thus listing in writing what was expected of the employee and the employer. This added a level of objectivity which had not previously existed. Further revisions have been made based on our realization of changes in the needs of both personnel and the setting.

By August of 1974 one unit—ICU-CCU—was being scheduled by the head nurse. The unit felt strongly that this was the method of scheduling they preferred. The nursing service office was used on a consultative basis to assist in problem solving and on an ancillary basis when additional staff was needed due to increase in census, staff vacations, illness, etc.

ATTITUDES DIFFER

The attitude of the unit in which staffing was decentralized was quite different from units in which centralized staffing was implemented. There was a marked increase in the sense of cohesiveness and responsibility exhibited by the decentralized unit. Gradually other units expressed a desire for some form of decentralized staffing. Usually the nurses on the unit are scheduled by a method of decentralized staffing and the unit clerks and family care assistants are scheduled through the staffing office. Variations of decentralized staffing have evolved, such as self staffing,

cyclical staffing or staffing by a staff member on the unit.

Role of Administrative Assistant for Staffing

As staffing has decentralized, the role of the administrative assistant for staffing has evolved from that of scheduler to communicator and coordinator. There is greater need for coordinating activities of staffing to meet patient care needs when decentralized staffing is used. The more diffused the staffing responsibilities, the more imperative communication becomes

The more diffused the staffing responsibilities, the more imperative communication becomes between the units and the nursing service office to assure that both the unit and the nursing office have an accurate record of the staff on duty and the projected schedules.

between the units and the nursing service office to assure that both the unit and nursing office have an accurate record of the staff on duty and the projected schedules. A breakdown in communications between the unit and office in this setting can produce problems in accurate payment of benefits and time worked.

The person presently functioning in the role has a social work background and consequently a natural tendency has been toward utilization of those skills in advising supervisory personnel, in working through situations with employees and in direct counseling with personnel to assist them in working through problems. The availability of a resource person with a social service background is valuable in that the employees' problems have ramifications affecting attendance and productivity. A person who is knowledgeable regarding social resources in the community expedites action on problems affecting the employees' work. Definition of the problem allows the employer to discuss possible alternatives of hours and positions that might be available in the setting which would be realistic and productive to both hospital and employee in light of the individual situation.

WORKING RELATIONSHIPS

It is important that a close working relationship exists between the director of nursing and the administrative assistant for staffing. The director of nursing provides guidance and input based on an overall perspective of the community, the hospital and interdepartmental relationships. It is essential that the director of nursing work closely with the people in the staffing office to provide direction for nursing care programs evolved from the hospital's philosophy.

The Staffing Office

There are a number of areas of responsibility that naturally fall into the realm of the staffing office. A major area of concern in health care today is

fiscal management, particularly living within the manpower budget. At Family Hospital the budget is monitored on a daily basis by patient care hours. We have found a job position control form which uses our patient care hour ratio, average census and also takes into account other variables which would affect manpower needs. This report gives an overview of what the average manpower needs are versus the actual number of personnel employed, both by classification and unit. This tool is invaluable in planning for recruitment and maintaining the budget. It is also helpful in objectively indicating the distribution of staff to the units. The job position control is maintained by the staffing office.

As personnel are needed, the personnel department is notified and the recruitment process is initiated. The nonprofessional staff such as clerical staff, unit clerks and family care assistants are hired by the administrative assistant for staffing. The professional nursing staff is interviewed and hired by the director of nursing.

Disciplinary action regarding atten-

The liaison activities between the nursing service office and personnel department are varied. However, the coordinating of these activities with one person eliminates overlapping of duties and reduces the chance of error or oversight.

dance problems is often initiated through the staffing office, although this is not an exclusive function of the office and may be initiated by an employee's clinical director. It has been our experience that corroboration with the personnel department prior to taking disciplinary action has been of great assistance in assuring that the approach taken is the most effective, as well as the most legally sound in light of labor relations legislation.

The liaison activities between the nursing service office and personnel department are varied. However, coordinating these activities with one person eliminates overlapping of duties and reduces the chance of error or oversight.

Communication Patterns

It is important that communication patterns be set which allow the employees the latitude to freely discuss concerns they may have with the administrative staff. It has been my experience that new graduates coming into the setting have unrealistic expectations as to the norm regarding staffing and nursing policies. This is coupled with the fact that their anxiety level is high, therefore, the need for effective communication is intensified.

The persons in the staffing office have daily contact with staff, and their ability to communicate on an objective basis is imperative. The role of the staffing manager is that of communicator and buffer between the nursing units, supervisors and other adminis-

trative personnel. The ability to transmit decisions and the rationale behind those decisions in an objective manner alerts the staff to the needs of other areas in the hospital.

SENSITIVITY TO NEEDS

Along with the ability to communicate effectively with staff, the nursing manager must be sensitive to the needs of the nursing staff, realizing when an employee has indicated that a level of satiation has been reached. Sensitivity to where an employee "is at" will keep us from abusing responsive employees by continually tapping them when staffing is short.

SHOWING APPRECIATION

Because these employees are responsive to the hospital's needs, the staffing manager must be aware of the danger of burn out. This can be avoided by responding to nonverbal messages indicating a need for a day off. A gentle approach in requesting extra time from personnel is imperative and it must be realized that everything beyond the hours these employees have committed themselves to is in a sense a gift of themselves, not something employers should view as their right. When appreciation for extra time worked is projected, employees experience the recognition of the dedication to the setting's needs and morale is kept up. When the feeling that overtime is owed to the institution is projected, defenses are raised and staffing managers' actions are self-defeating.

INVOLVEMENT OF NONNURSE PERSONNEL

The involvement of a professional person with a background other than nursing (in our case, a social worker) has advantages which have been tapped in the setting at Family Hospital. The obvious advantage is that in an area suffering from a shortage of nurses, placing another professional in staffing frees a nurse for patient care. A less obvious benefit is that the nonnurse brings another perspective to the administrative staff. Such an eclectic approach should broaden the outlook of the group in dealing with the concerns of the department.

The role of the person in charge of a staffing office is that of facilitator, advisor, coordinator and liaison. The strongest component needed for the successful completion of the duties of the position is the ability to communicate—to both give and receive messages, attitudes and philosophies. The philosophy this person has regarding the dignity and worth of the individual will permeate the manner of communication; consequently, it is important that the values this person places on the individual be consistent with the value system of the institution.

Anne M. Harvieux, B.A., Sociology
Administrative Assistant
for Staffing
Family Hospital

HOSPITAL SERVICE ASSISTANT—A NEW ROLE IN NURSING SERVICES

111

Two years ago, the P.M. nursing supervisor at Family Hospital would have had to obtain Gomco suctions, cold steamers and a variety of other central supply items. After eight P.M., nursing supervisors prepared meals and nourishments, plus made an occasional trip to central stores for items not on the nursing units. If a floor ran out of linen, you know who had to go to the linen room.

One of the most time-consuming tasks for both the personnel on the nursing units as well as the supervisor was transporting patients from admitting to their rooms. Also, patients had to be taken to the laboratory, x-ray and other departments. Not only did nursing supervisors have to take the individual to the various departments, they also had to stay with the patient. Often more time was spent carrying out these nonnursing functions than performing the higher priority items listed in our job description for nursing supervisors.

In 1975 we participated in a leadership effectiveness training course conducted at Family Hospital. The course participants included several department heads as well as leaders in nursing service. One of our course projects was to identify a problem area and try to resolve it. The problem that we felt was most important for P.M.s, particularly on weekends when staffing was short, was a lack of personnel available to transport patients from admitting to the laboratory, x-ray and nursing units. We found several other department members concerned and involved in our problem as it interfaced with their departments.

Finding a Solution

Our group generated 17 different possible solutions to this problem. In prioritizing the alternatives, the group determined the need to create a new position to be filled by a former nursing assistant who would basically serve as a transportation aide. The function of the person in this new position would be to transport patients coming to and leaving ancillary departments and assist patients in these areas.

For a two-month period we gathered statistics that proved nursing service lost 140 minutes a night in the transportation of patients for x-ray. We concluded we would need someone who would be available not only to handle transportation to and from the x-ray department, but to and from other departments as well.

After our two-month statistic-gathering period, we shared our findings with nursing administration and a position was allocated on the budget.

Our next step was to present our position proposal to the hospital administrator. Our group presented the problem to him as well as our solution. He was supportive of this, so we then developed the job description. It was agreed that experienced nursing assistants would be best qualified for

the job because they could help on the nursing units when not busy. Two experienced nursing assistants volunteered for the position, and together they have expanded their role to what is presently our hospital service assistant. Under the direction of the nursing administrative supervisor, the hospital service assistant's duties consist of the following:

1. Transport and assist patients from nursing units to service departments, i.e., radiology, laboratory, out-patient, admitting, pre-op classes, etc. and return patients to their rooms.
2. Assist patients while in service departments as necessary.
3. Collect and distribute requisitions, reports, specimens, supplies, flowers, etc. between service departments and nursing units.
4. Assist with food distribution for patients and employees.
5. Perform nursing assistant duties such as answering call lights, feeding patients, assisting patients with their personal needs, take temperature, pulse, respiration.
6. Perform other related duties as assigned.

Because two people fill this position, we have seven day coverage. When the hospital service assistants report to work, they pick up a pager to be readily accessible to anyone in the hospital who would need their services. They also are assigned to a nursing unit to help out when not busy, which is very seldom.

113

The role of the hospital service assistant has proved to be a tremendous help to us as supervisors, because it has relieved us of many nonnursing tasks. We are now able to spend more time with staff on the nursing units and in other administrative functions.

The role of the hospital service assistant has proved to be a tremendous help to us as supervisors, because it has relieved us of many nonnursing tasks. We are now able to spend more time with the staff on the nursing units and in other administrative functions.

In addition to being a great assist to the supervisors, the hospital service assistant's role has helped facilitate family-centered care by freeing the nurses of many of these nonnursing duties. This means better utilization of everyone's time with patients and more time for clinical consultation.

David Falk, R.N.
Marion Muscavitch, R.N.
P.M. Supervisors
Family Hospital

NURSE RECRUITMENT

What approach may be used to attract new graduates to a private community hospital in a large city already suffering from a severe shortage of nurses?

The graduate nurses of today are approaching their potential job market with an even greater understanding of the different components that contribute to the total employment picture. Because these graduates have sorted out their priorities in searching for an employer, the sophistication in which they are approached continues to become a more important element of the total recruitment process.

Team Effort

It has been our experience that the nursing service department alone cannot be expected to assume the total role of nurse recruitment. A partnership which includes direct input from nursing service, personnel and administration can contribute significantly as a total team effort. It is an effort that is adapted to most effectively handle the different areas of inquiry, from nursing philosophy, histories and care plans to monetary considerations, employee benefits and additional fringes that make up the total employee offering.

In this team effort, each department participates, offering its particular expertise. Time is devoted to concentrate on answers to specific questions graduate nurses have regarding each specialty area.

The Nurse Recruiter

A nurse recruiter is vital in attracting nurses to our hospital. Having a professional background is necessary in relating to nursing and the patient care situation. Enthusiasm and a commitment to the philosophy of the hos-

114

pital has been an important factor in the total interpersonal relationship while interviewing the graduate nurse. If the nurse recruiter is enthusiastic and excited about the progressive nursing care system, graduate nurses are more than likely to show some interest as they discover a hospital practicing nursing the way they have been taught.

There must be a catch! When touring the facility with the graduates, I encourage them to relate to a staff nurse who has recently completed our nurse internship program. Arrangements are available for nurses to spend a morning observing a family care nurse in action. Seeing is believing.

My role as nurse recruiter has been primarily to interview and give graduate nurses a tour of the facilities. During the interview and general discussion, I find myself focusing on the hospital philosophy. This gives graduate nurses a good idea as to where administration is coming from regarding their commitment to the health care delivery system. Nurses want to know if the system is compatible with their professional goals.

Primary nursing or family-centered care nursing is another aspect that is covered and explained in depth. Unfortunately, the semantics of primary nursing are misleading, and it is my responsibility to explain exactly what an individual's role as family care nurse would be. Each graduate nurse is provided with a complete job description of the staff position. At this time our goal is to select nurses

> *The semantics of primary nursing are misleading . . . each graduate nurse is provided with a complete job description of the staff position . . . our goal is to select nurses who are compatible with our professional role expectations.*

who are compatible with our professional role expectations.

The three-month nurse internship program and its components are discussed in greater detail, for this orientation program is vital to newly graduated nurses today as they make the transition from graduate nurses to RNs.

I have also found it important to focus upon the progressive programs unique to Family Hospital, such as nursing research, the sexual assault treatment center and patient teaching. Progressive graduate nurses are most likely attracted to those things that other hospitals are unable to offer.

Certainly the team effort has afforded an interdependence that has led to success. Each component is vital and invaluable to an effective recruitment program.

Judy Jahde, R.N.
Nurse Recruiter
Family Hospital

An Employment Supervisor

It has been our experience that there is a very distinct advantage in including a representative of the personnel department in the total process of interviewing the new graduates. In my role as employment supervisor, I related with professional personnel interpretation the specifics of pay, raises, vacations, sick days, insurances and other employee fringes to the candidates. The highlights of each benefit can be emphasized in order to "sell" the attractive and total employee benefit package.

In addition, the personnel function can contribute significantly after the actual interview process has been completed. The total processing of the application including securing references and transcripts, coordinating the pre-employment physical exam, setting up payroll paperwork and benefit enrollments, relieves the nursing department of this time-consuming paper processing.

Our personnel-nursing teamwork is equally as significant at state conven-

While emphasis may vary in each employment situation, it is important to recognize the key benefits of a total team effort . . . the interdependence of this team is our key to successful recruiting.

tions, career days and on-campus recruitment activities as it is in the active recruitment process.

While emphasis may vary in each employment situation, it is important to recognize the key benefits of a total team effort. It has been our experience that the interdependence of this team is our key to successful recruiting.

MariKay Bruno
Employment Supervisor
Family Hospital

A Penetration Coefficient Approach to Nursing Staffing

Thomas R. O'Donovan, Ph.D.
Administrator
Mt. Carmel Mercy Hospital
Detroit, Michigan

A PENETRATION COEFFICIENT approach to nursing staffing assists in determining proper staffing levels for any unit within any hospital. Even though it often happens in staffing that employment of "all who can be obtained" still results in short staffing, we will assume that by taking a proper and realistic approach to staffing determination we can augment occasional short staffing by strategic planning.

Hospitals occasionally overstaff on some shifts in some units and understaff in others. When this happens we always hear about the understaffing but never the overstaffing. Of course, the greater problem is how do you know when you are over or understaffed, and when you do know, who will agree with that analysis?

Certain assumptions have been made in this approach, which will be described later, and a product of these assumptions, a nursing service staffing . . . penetration coefficient . . . will be derived for all units. This

118

> *Hospitals occasionally overstaff on some shifts in some units and understaff in others. When this happens we always hear about the understaffing but never the overstaffing.*

assists us in preparing an approach to staffing. It will be difficult to obtain all-pervasive criteria. Since it cannot be done statistically, it has to be done on the basis of utilization of competent judgment by people who know nursing well, and by evaluating staffing levels achieved under this type of system. The wisdom and judgment of administrators, directors of nursing service, assistant directors and supervisors, both floor supervisors and shift supervisors, is essential.

STATISTICAL APPROACH HAS PROBLEMS

It should be noted at the onset that there are many problems involved in taking a statistical approach. Nevertheless, we should attempt the task in the hope of shedding light so that staffing decisions can be made on a more sound basis than guesswork, hunch or past experience.

In deriving such an approach, we must assign certain values to differing classifications of personnel. If we attempt to grade these individuals as to their flexibility and utilization, the best approach is normally a complete review of a job description to de-

termine the functional responsibility of each classification. For the purpose of this presentation, note that we have assigned an index value of one to RNs, .75 to LPNs and .50 to aides. These figures are based upon how much or what duties can be performed by RNs which cannot be performed by LPNs or aides. Similarly, what duties can be performed by LPNs which cannot be performed by aides. The actual functional responsibilities in each hospital would determine, or would at least assist in determining, what values would be placed on each classification of personnel.

The major point is that it is *not* realistic to assume that all nursing personnel classifications "penetrate" patient care the same way. Ratios of 4.5 hours of care provide a consistent comparison from unit to unit or hospital to hospital *as far as numbers go,* but what if two units of the same size have the following total staffing complement:

	Unit 1	Unit 2
RN	2	10
LPN	3	0
Aide	5	0
	10	10

Can we really say that the staffing is identical here? These units may have 4.5 or some such statistical norm, but are they truly similar? Assigning differential coefficients helps relate units, shifts and even hospitals to one another more realistically! (See Table 1.)

TABLE 1
Conventional vs Penetration Coefficient Staffing Methods

Conventional Method:

	Days	Afternoons	Midnights	Total	
RN	2	1	1	4	
LPN	3	2	1	6	$\dfrac{18 \times 24 \text{ hrs}}{3 \times 30 = 90} = 4.8$
Aides, Orderlies, Unit Clerks	5	2	1	8	
Total	10	5	3	18	

Average Census: 30 30 30

Staffing ratio for 24 hour day: 4.8

$$\begin{array}{r} 4.8 \\ 90\overline{)432.} \\ \underline{360} \\ 72 \end{array}$$

Proposed Method:

	Days	P.C.	Afternoons	P.C.	Midnights	P.C.	Total P.C.
RN	2	2	1	1	1	1	4
LPN	3	2.25	2	1.5	1	.75	4.5
Aides, Orderlies, Unit Clerks	5	2.5	2	1	1	.50	4.0
Total		6.75		3.5		2.25	12.5

Average Census 30 30 30

Formula: $\dfrac{\text{P.C. } (12.5) \times 24 \text{ hrs}}{90} = 3.3$

Thus, a 4.8 becomes a 3.3, which is the more valid penetration of care to patients.

Factors Affecting the Penetration Coefficient

ASSIGNING INDEX NUMBERS

In assigning index numbers to occupational groups, there are many shortcomings. Included among these are:

- In some units, such as geriatrics, LPNs may be equal to RNs in the patient care being extended. This means that the relationships between RNs, LPNs and aides might be a function of the type of unit we are discussing, rather than the job classifications per se.
- The mix is vital. Until the basic needs are met, LPNs cannot be substituted for RNs on a .75 to one basis. After basic staffing patterns have been obtained, adding an LPN might be more important than adding an RN.
- The rating of the job classifications as one, .75 or .50 is merely an estimate that may never be statistically proven either correct or *incorrect*. The contribution and competency of people vary so much that it would not be useful to "overanalyze" the data. Rating people might result in a range from one-sixteenth to five. Then

120

what do we do with our neat array of statistical charts, graphs and tables?

BALANCE OF INDEX NUMBERS

If no RN is available, adding ten aides will not achieve good patient care. Therefore, the index value of one for RNs, .75 for LPNs, and .50 for aides and orderlies must be balanced. The LPN total may be less than the RN total, and the aide and orderly total may best be above the RN total in some instances, and lower in other situations.

EVALUATING HEAD NURSES

A question arises as to how much evaluation head nurses could receive in relation to the nurses that are assigned to the general duty care. If head nurses perform only managerial duties and activities not related to direct patient care, they should count zero in computing staffing levels. Because of the several reasons about to be mentioned, it may be useful to assign a value of .75 to head nurses. The reasons that complicate the issue as to the assigning of an index of service given to head nurses are:

- Staffing levels may be short one day and adequate the next day, which means that head nurses will be performing more general staff nursing duties on days when they are short staffed, and head nurse duties when they are adequately staffed.
- Float personnel assigned to their units may not be as useful as their regular personnel, which increases the head nurses' involvement. Newly-assigned personnel fresh out of a two-year program will not be as useful as experienced regular personnel.
- The value system of individual head nurses themselves may be such that they lean to general nursing duties more than to the executive activities necessary in the job.
- A consistent short staffing of nursing personnel on the unit and a lack of messenger service, desk clerks, etc., may result in the head nurses' inability to function as they need to.
- Even though head nurses spend most of their time in leadership activities rather than general nursing activities, assigning them a .75 can be partially justified by the fact that general staff nurses are given a general index of one even though they may be part of a team nursing system and perform much of their duties as team leaders rather than as general duty nurses.

Of course, the secret to all this is universal acceptance so that all hospitals use the same approach, otherwise we could never compare them.

If head nurses perform only managerial duties and activities not related to direct patient care, they should count zero in computing staffing levels.

The objective of assigning these classifications to personnel is to arrive at a total number of "penetration coefficients" which is needed in each unit. If a penetration coefficient number is four on the day shift of three Main, this number could possibly be composed of two RNs, two LPNs and one aide. Or, depending upon the hospital's needs, which will be defined in the considerations involved later, it might be one RN and four LPNs, or other formulations.

PROBLEMS OF COMPARISON

This brings us to some of the problems with comparing the statistical approach among hospitals and their staffing, and even among units of an existing hospital. Some of these problems are included in the following list:

- How well are the patients? New surgical patients require more care than do third or fourth day surgical cases, and chronic cases may have great dependency without being too ill. The **degree of illness** on each unit is a major determinant in basic staffing needs. Unless this is known, we cannot statistically compare the staffing needs of one unit or hospital to another.
- **What types of patients are being cared for?** The difference in the type and amount of care exists between medical, surgical, obstetric, ICU, pediatric, etc., patients.
- **How consistent is the census?** In some of the services mentioned

Under certain circumstances, the greater the total square footage of a nursing unit, the greater the staffing needs, if the number of patients is held constant.

above, particularly pediatrics and obstetrics, we see great fluctuations in the census. Staffing these units is particularly difficult when trying to use statistical methods.

- **What is the layout of each unit?** Are there special arrangements on specific units? How far do personnel have to walk to get supplies and equipment and to observe patients?
- **How much automation is there on each unit?** Does each unit have, for example, bedpan washers, ice-makers, nurse call intercommunication to patients?
- **Are medications centralized or decentralized** from the pharmacy? Do we have a traditional medication system or a unit-dose system?
- **What types of rooms are there on each unit**—ward, semi, or private? What is the mix of these types of rooms on each unit? Although patients are often deprived of privacy in ward units, many nurses would comment that the nursing care time in terms of personal services to patients is increased in a ward simply by the proximity of each patient to the nurse. Under certain circumstances, the greater the total

NURSE STAFFING

122

square footage of a nursing unit, the greater the staffing needs, if the number of patients is held constant.

- **What type of bathroom facilities are there for patients?** Are there separate bathrooms or toilets for each room? Are there handwashing facilities in each room? If not, a great deal of wasted time is incurred while nursing staff wash between treating each patient, or when they are required to accompany patients to bathrooms outside their individual rooms.
- **Are disposables used** and to what extent?
- **Is there clerical staffing,** and is the desk clerk trained and available for one shift, two shifts or three shifts? To what extent is this clerk trained, and does it relieve the floor nurses of a great deal of time spent in nonnursing tasks?
- **Are unit managers being used?** What are the total responsibilities of the head nurses? Do they do the unit staffing themselves or does the nursing office perform this function? (All three of these factors affect comparative differentiations.)
- **Which shift is being considered?** Day and afternoon staffing should definitely be greater than night staffing, and what ratio is considered appropriate among each of the three shifts?
- **What are the job descriptions for the nursing personnel?** Do LPNs give medications? What is the meeting and conference schedule

of the personnel on this unit? Are float nurses available for absenteeism? Does the hospital occasionally use an outside medical pool when short-run needs dictate?

- **Is team nursing utilized?** This particular method normally requires more staffing.
- Regarding administrative philosophy, **does the administration of the hospital desire or require a nearly all RN staff?**
- **Are patients truly separated?** Does the admitting office keep medical patients out of surgical areas (and vice versa)?
- **Is there an overall reluctance by the nursing service personnel to float from unit to unit?** Or from shift to shift? The index number approach takes large areas into consideration, but it doesn't assist if a particular area is short.
- **The managerial ability of each head nurse** affects the staffing and the efficiency on each unit.
- **The ratio of staffing on days, afternoons and midnights** is interrelated. Higher staffing on afternoons may be justified if nights are extremely short staffed. The patients can be settled better by leaving high staffing on afternoons. A ratio of 100 percent staffing on days, 70 percent staffing on afternoons and 30 percent staffing on nights could go to 100, 95, 20, simply because of the night short staffing.
- **The difference between units** can be exemplified by the ICU theory

that the staffing ratio over days, afternoons and midnights would be 100, 100, 100. But because more doctors are around on *days* and they need attention, and the nurses must be available to attend to the orders of the physicians, assist with tests, treatments, dressings and physical examinations, the theory of 100, 100, 100 could possibly be modified to 100, 80, 80. (This point needs further study as to its applicability to the medical/surgical units, etc.)

- **Are many versus few private duty nurses utilized?** Are student nurses used extensively throughout the hospital? Does the hospital have a good volunteer force which assists the nursing service department? These kinds of points affect differential staffing patterns.
- **Policies on linen exchange, leaving the nursing station, patient transportation,** and simply whether or not messenger services are available, play a large part in staffing analysis.
- **The extent of a high degree of specialization** results occasionally in certain nurses being idle in their specialty unit, while nurses in other units are temporarily highly involved or short of help. The problem is how to maximize the advantages of nurse specialization and still have the effective use of them in slack periods. Where feasible, nurses could be trained in two or three specialized areas so that flexibility can be achieved. (PAR, ICU, OB, ER, etc.)

- **Differential ability and levels of training among nursing personnel** must be considered. The individual nurse competency is a highly relevant issue. (This makes it very difficult to apply arbitrary statistical measures to staffing determinations.)
- **The size of the medical staff** is certainly an issue at hand. Those hospitals with large medical staffs may find they need more nurses to handle the physicians' orders. Those hospitals with small medical staffs may find that nurses have assumed more and more of the physicians' duties.
- **The fringe benefit package at the hospital** must be considered. Do employees after five years receive four weeks' vacation, three weeks, one week? Do "all" employees after five years receive four weeks' vacation? Since fringe benefit policies, particularly vacation, holiday and sick day policies, relate to the hours of each employee throughout a year, the numbers of personnel assigned to each unit are directly

---

Those hospitals with large medical staffs may find they need more nurses to handle the physicians' orders. Those hospitals with small medical staffs may find that nurses have assumed more and more of the physicians' duties.

124

affected by these policies. How many coffee breaks are allowed, and how long, and does abuse exist?

So many short-run variables affect staffing determinations that it is simply not realistic to apply rigid requirements to all units within any hospital.

However, as long as we are truly aware of all the above mentioned factors, it makes good sense to plan all staffing patterns based on sound judgment and assign nursing personnel accordingly! Haphazard staffing determinations are unnecessarily expensive. There is no substitute for good planning. The framework presented herein needs much further study and can form the springboard for sound research into the mystery of attaining optimum staffing patterns in any health care facility.

Nurse Staffing in the Context of Institutional and State-Level Planning

Mary Segall, R.N., Ph.D.
Associate Professor
University of Colorado
School of Nursing
Denver, Colorado

Ken Sauer, M.S.
Senior Staff Associate
National Center for Higher
Education Management Systems
Boulder, Colorado

In considering staffing questions, nursing administrators are likely to focus on the number and type of nursing personnel needed for a particular unit, institution or agency. And rightly so, since staffing questions are crucial to the kind of care being provided to their patients. But in a time when planning strategies and regulatory measures are receiving considerable attention in the health care industry, it increasingly is in the interest of nursing administrators to broaden their perspectives to include considerations that extend beyond institutional boundaries when addressing staffing and program development needs. A perspective that focuses primarily on one's own institution neglects the dynamic interplay between forces—such as the educa-

This article resulted from a project, "Analysis and Planning for Improved Distribution of Nursing Personnel and Services," undertaken under HEW, Division of Nursing, Contract #231-75-0803, with the Western Interstate Commission for Higher Education and the National Center for Higher Education Management Systems, Boulder, Colorado.

126 tion systems, the health planning community and consumer perferences—which influence the availability and utilization of nursing personnel.

While there is a relatively rich literature on institutional staffing approaches, there is a need for material describing state-level manpower planning methodologies. Although more than enough has been written which describes and summarizes the National Health Planning and Resources Development Act of 1974 (PL 93-641), what has not been adequately addressed are the substantive issues that planners must grapple with in attempting to implement the law and plan at the state or HSA level. (The term *state* in this article includes substate regions such as the Health Service Areas (HSAs) and groupings of counties.) For example, precisely how does one go about estimating future health manpower needs and resources for a state? What planning methodologies are available to assist in making those projections? Whose expertise should be called upon to evaluate and modify the projections? What data can one use? Nurses must

---

Nurses must do more than be appointed to the advisory boards of the Health Systems Agencies—they must also be conversant with planning language and concepts so that they are able to participate more fully and substantively in the planning process.

---

do more than be appointed to the advisory boards of the Health Systems Agencies—they must also be conversant with planning language and concepts so that they are able to participate more fully and substantively in the planning process.

NEED FOR EXTRA-INSTITUTIONAL PERSPECTIVE

Nursing administrators are concerned about the nursing needs of their clients within their institutions. They are equally concerned about participating in some kind of a system of coordination of client care that extends beyond their institutional boundaries of jurisdiction. However, this duality of concern frequently has not been evidenced in planning for staffing.

In Aydelotte's review of the literature concerning staffing, several predominant themes emerge: the measurement of nursing productivity; the quality of nursing care provided to clients; patient classification schemes; organization of nursing personnel within units (for example, team versus primary nursing); and various methodologies drawn from operations research and industrial engineering to determine staffing assignments.[1]

This literature suggests a concern primarily with the institutional aspects of staffing. However, there are other responsibilities—for the most part patient-related—currently carried out by nursing administrators that are extra-institutional in nature. For example, nursing administrators participate and are concerned about developing a coordinated system of alternatives for care of patients discharged from a hospital. These alternatives may include linkages with nursing homes, home care support services and ambulatory clinics. Although nursing administrators participate in extra-institutional as well as intra-institutional planning for patient-related purposes, we feel there is little extra-institutional planning with regard to staffing.

Incentives

However, there are incentives for becoming involved with staffing issues beyond the immediate institutional considerations. For example, there are a number of legislative imperatives which call for a wider involvement in staffing planning. The long-range plans and annual implementation plans specified under PL 93-641 contain provisions that have definite effects on manpower and staffing questions. Similarly, the certificate-of-need concept as embodied in Section 1122 of the amendments to the Social Security Act requires that the plans for the construction of new facilities or the expansion of existing ones be reviewed by an officially designated planning agency. What is important to note is that one component of the review is to include consideration of the question of how the new or expanded facility can be staffed. Finally, Part D of the Nurse Training Act of 1975 (PL 94-63) calls for the supply, distribution and requirements of nurses to be determined for each of the states.

Planning

127

Although current legislation provides clear evidence of the trend toward manpower and staff planning at the state level, why should nursing administrators become involved in such planning efforts? There seem to be at least two responses to that question. Planning decisions made at the state level are going to affect the amount, type and placement of health care programs available within the health care delivery system which will in turn impact the staffing needs of particular institutions. Planning decisions also will be made which will influence the number and educational preparation of nursing personnel who are available to meet the staffing needs of a given institution. Given the involvement of nursing administrators with nursing services being provided and the staff required to provide those services, they are an excellent resource to provide direction for nursing manpower planning done at the state level.

DIFFERENCES BETWEEN STATE-LEVEL AND INSTITUTIONAL PLANNING

As was indicated previously, nursing administrators must be conversant with planning concepts and perspectives. Planning for nurse staffing at the institutional level as compared to the state level deals with different sets of concerns and issues. The differences can be identified as follows: at the state level (1) the concerns seem to be broader and more complex since the *focus* of planning is different; (2)

128

multiple *options* exist with respect to programs and personnel; (3) more people with varying *perspectives* are involved in the decision-making process; (4) the *time frame* is longer; and (5) collection of and access to *data* is exceedingly cumbersome. Understanding some of these differences should facilitate nursing administrators' effective participation in planning and influencing change at the state level.

Focus

The focus in planning the delivery of health care at the state level is on groups of people rather than specific individuals. As an example, when focusing on groups, one utilizes statistical rates of the incidence of diseases to develop plans for intervention, in contrast to working with particular individuals and their individual, unique health problems. The criteria for evaluation of the delivery of care are similar when planning at both the institutional and state levels; that is, administrators at each of these levels are concerned about access, availability, quality and cost effectiveness of nursing care. However, at the state level the objective is to meet these criteria in relation to groups and at the institutional level in relation to specific individuals.

The example of a specialized critical care unit may serve to illustrate the differences in terms of focus between the institutional and state-level perspectives. At the institutional level, administrators are concerned that the clients have a direct and clear route of referral to the critical care unit from various health care providers. They should not have to wait too long or travel too far and should receive cost effective quality care. By way of contrast, state-level concerns include estimating how many people would require and utilize critical care units; where the units should be located in terms of distance to the population with the highest risk; and how many nursing personnel are available or could be attracted to staff these units.

Options

A second difference between the state and institutional perspective relates to whether or not the health care delivery system for the state is considered in its entirety. Generally, institutional administrators are concerned with the efficient and effective operation of the agency, particularly in relation to coordination of programs and staff within the agency, although some effort may be directed toward coordination with other components that directly interface with their own institution and their clients' needs. As an example, nursing administrators of a hospital may arrange for home care of discharged patients through the services of a visiting nursing agency.

However, at the state level, planning for all the components of the delivery system must be considered. When this consideration is given, multiple options for planning can be developed in relation to alternative ways of delivering health care services, varying staffing patterns utilizing different types of health care providers, and differing arrangements for reimbursement in order to meet the health needs of the population. It is unlikely that a plan with this kind of flexibility in terms of programming, providers and reimbursement mechanisms could be orchestrated at the institutional level.

Perspectives

A third difference between institutional and state-level planning is the number and diversity of groups involved in the decision-making process. At the institutional level, nursing administrators gain experience in understanding the perspectives of hospital administrators, other service directors within the agency and the agency executive board. However, at the state level different groups of people, with whom nursing administrators may not have had experience in interacting, participate in developing or approving plans for nursing manpower. The groups of people and interests which they represent may be characterized in

At the institutional level, nursing administrators gain experience in understanding the perspectives of hospital administrators, other service directors within the agency and the agency executive board ... at the state level different groups of people participate in developing or approving plans for nursing manpower.

the following way:

- The **health professions group** includes nurses, physicians, other health professionals and representatives of state nursing associations and regulatory agencies. Their perspective is to provide the very best care that is possible for those individuals who present themselves for care.
- The **health planning group** includes state health officials, hospital administrators, health economists and members of Health Systems Agencies. This group's priority concerns are allocation of money and manpower resources which will do the most good for the most people.
- The **higher education group** includes the state coordinating/governing board of postsecondary education and deans of schools of nursing. Deans frequently have as their goal increasing enrollment and offering a diversity of educational programs. The state coordinating boards are faced with responding to the needs of the nursing education sector as well as the requests from all other education programs.
- The **legislative group** includes state legislators whose decisions influence planning priorities and budgetary matters. The legislative community is besieged by multiple pressures and requests. Although individual legislators' jobs are to represent the interests of their constituents in order to be

130

reelected, as a group, legislators approve the budget and formulate policy. Usually legislative joint budget committees will not have health interests as a major priority.

Given that the perspectives and responsibilities of each of these groups are different, one can appreciate the kind of arena in which nursing administrators will be participating. One can also understand the politics which influence the development of consensus around a state-wide health plan which would be credible to the various groups. Reaching consensus is indeed necessary in order for a health plan to be workable and credible to the groups involved. The tactics of negotiation and bargaining to influence a health plan at the state level are different and less familiar to nursing administrators than the tactics used to influence others within their own institutions.

Time Frame

A fourth difference between institutional and state-level planning is that the time frame for planning at the state level is usually longer than it is for institutional planning. At the institutional level the time frame for planning for staffing needs ranges from immediate day-to-day needs to longer range concerns that are usually up to a year. Day-to-day staffing concerns are exemplified by determining who is working a particular shift or responsible for a group of clients. An example of intermediate institutional staffing concerns is hiring additional staff. If a

new position in nursing has been approved, the normal expectation is that a person would be hired within several months. Long-range institutional planning is typified by nursing administrators who prepare a budget for staffing and program needs for the forthcoming year.

In contrast to the institution, the time frame for planning at the state level is rarely less than a year and frequently extends to five or more years. For example, if there is a consensus that the state needs to increase the number of nurses with a master's degree in nursing, one or more graduate nursing programs may be needed. Initiation of a graduate nursing educational program generally requires one or more years. It takes time to develop the curriculum, recruit qualified faculty and identify clinical laboratory facilities. Thus, the immediate effect will not be realized for several years, and the full impact of the graduates from the program will not be felt for probably a decade.

Data

Data issues are highlighted here because of the importance that data have for use in decision making. At the institutional level, nursing administrators have control over and are able to collect the needed data from the particular institution. In collecting the data, institutional administrators do not need to worry about collecting data according to a common set of definitions in order to have comparable data among other institutions. In contrast, the lack of a framework for collecting comparable health-related data among institutions is a major problem at the state level. In institutional planning less data are required; the data are collected from fewer sources and more easily analyzed than data needed for a state nursing plan.

Given the breadth of issues and concerns in nursing manpower planning at the state level and the multiplicity of perspectives and persons involved in decision making, it is apparent that both the methodology and process used for state planning will need to be different than that used at the institutional level.

AN APPROACH FOR ESTIMATING NURSING REQUIREMENTS

A model for estimating nursing personnel requirements is presented in Figure 1. The term *requirements* refers to the number of nursing personnel that will be needed to meet a particular set of health care goals. The model consists of three components: a requirements planning process, a data base to facilitate the planning process and a set of mathematical equations for estimating state-level projections of nurses needed.

The relationships between the components can be described in the following way. Planners and participants would first proceed through the steps in the requirements planning process and address the planning questions raised in the process. Recent data is referred to in addressing the questions. After full consideration of the questions raised in going through the planning process, the participants then make certain assumptions about such areas as changes in the health care delivery system, in staffing patterns and utilization over

131

FIGURE 1. MODEL FOR ESTIMATING NURSING REQUIREMENTS: STEPS IN REQUIREMENTS PLANNING PROCESS

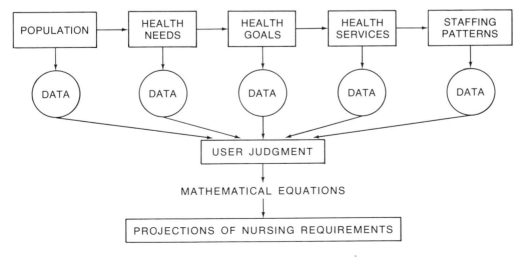

132

the next five years. These professional judgments are used as input in computing the mathematical equations to make projections about the number and types of nurses needed in the future. An overview of the steps in the requirements planning process follows.[2]

Differentiating the Population

The first decision point in the requirements planning process involves examining the population that is being and will be served rather than starting from the perspective of the institution delivering services. Data on such demographic variables as age, sex, race/ethnicity, income, educational attainment and occupation have been documented in the research literature as affecting both the population's need for and utilization of health care services.[3, 4, 5, 6] By examining readily available census data and other data which differentiates the population for a particular locality, such as the health service area, it is possible to gain greater insight into the health needs of the population. Examples which illustrate this point are:

- Morbidity/mortality rates will differ with respect to the age, sex and ethnic distribution of the population.
- Occupational differences also will account for morbidity/mortality discrepancies. Coal miners are susceptible to black lung disease, while office workers are prone to cardiovascular disease.

- Educational attainment affects personal health habits.

Examining Health Status Indicators

Closely related to generally differentiating the population is the next decision point: how to assess the health status of the population in terms of qualitative health status indicators. We have defined health status indicators as quantitative measures that directly or indirectly reflect the health of a given population. The concept of "good health" is proclaimed by various authors and organizations, but is difficult to measure and consequently difficult to determine if it is achieved or acquired. Given the problems of quantifying measures of the "healthy," numerical indicators most typically used are those which reflect who has died or been ill by the type or cause of the problem. Incidence and prevalence rates for certain communicable diseases, such as small pox and diphtheria, are rather systematically reported. However, similar types of morbidity data for noncommunicable diseases, such as cancer, diabetes or malnutrition, usually are collected only by means of special and infrequent surveys.

Indicators which measure numbers of days spent in bed, days lost from work or days absent from school may also be used. These types of data are suggestive of morbidity in the population at large, but are at best limited in their value since they are usually neither disease nor age and sex specific. It would be difficult to determine the type of specific health care programs that would be required or appropriate using this type of data.

Indirect health status indicators reflect data describing the environment in which people live and work which may exert an impact on health. Examples include measures of air quality and the safety of housing. Research studies suggest that air pollution does adversely affect the health of certain groups of the population, in particular elderly people with chronic respiratory diseases, such as emphysema and bronchitis.[7]

It is apparent that there are some complex planning problems associated with the measurement and collection of population-based health statistics. The use of these statistics is fraught with measurement and other types of data problems. However, to assume that the population of a particular locality is homogeneous with respect to its health care needs is, in effect, ignoring subsequent decisions that should be made with regard to the identification of needed programs and appropriate allocation of manpower.

Choosing Realizable Health Goals

The next decision point relates to the identification of a specific set of health goals, or if general health goals already exist, the adoption of these into a form which is usable for planning purposes. These goals will form the basis upon which subsequent decisions about health services and nursing utilization will be made.

133

Goals are important in that they represent a definition of problems to be solved for the well being of people in a particular area. A list of goals helps those involved in the planning process focus on defined problems.

Goals are important in that they represent a definition of problems to be solved for the well being of people in a particular area. A list of goals helps those involved in the planning process focus on defined problems. Without a clear statement of goals, discussion bogs down in needless arguments and mistaken assumptions. An agreed-upon set of goals, grouped according to priority, is essential to the plan.[8]

The process of formulating health goals should be influenced by the analysis of the population and their health needs. Also one might consider health goals that have been identified at the federal level. For example, in PL 93-641, ten national health priorities have been stated. Other sources to examine are goals stated by the governor's office or area-wide health planning agencies.

Developing a Health Strategy—Health Care Program and Services

Once the health goals have been determined, the question of programmatic thrusts should be considered. For the purpose of this project, the concept of program was defined as a particular combination of activities carried out to accomplish a particular

134 set of goals. Examples of health care programs are: inpatient, ambulatory, preventive, curative and tertiary care. Thus, the health care delivery system may be said to offer a number of health care programs.

In this project, we encountered the problem of the lack of a conceptual scheme for categorizing health care programs. We also would like to note the omission of *institutional* settings from the discussion of health care programs. This intentional omission of settings is intended to emphasize coordination and deemphasize fragmentation. This implies that planning should first deal with the thrust of the whole health care delivery system—the overall intended impact of the system—before dealing with more detailed consideration. Detailed planning without a master programmatic emphasis is more likely to result in less effective and duplicative outcomes. Thus, when operating at the programmatic level, the planner is not concerned with where health care services are institutionally housed; rather, the concern is with the overall effect of the services.

In considering which particular health care programs should be provided to achieve the health goals that have been developed, the following issues can be highlighted. Depending upon the emphasis various health care programs receive, an opportunity is available for changing the way in which the health care delivery system is structured. Second is the issue of cost containment. By shifting the existing relative emphasis of health programs, for example, from predominantly inpatient to an increase in ambulatory and outreach programs, it may be possible to achieve less costly health care with no loss in quality. Third, considerations of health programs may also underscore the importance of emphasizing wellness-oriented preventive care in health planning.

Determining Nursing Service Staffing

In the last step of the requirements planning process the focus is on staffing questions. After addressing staffing questions, one is in a position to begin the task of making quantitative nursing personnel projections.

Aydelotte clearly expressed her sentiments about nursing staffing methodology for practice settings. It should be an orderly, systematic process, based upon sound rationale, applied to determine the number and kinds of nursing personnel required to provide nursing care of a predetermined standard to a group of patients in a particular setting.[9]

Some of the questions about nursing staffing which need to be addressed are: How many direct client care RNs, LPNs and aides are needed for particular health care services? What are the educational preparations needed for direct client care RNs? How many administrative RNs are needed? What educational preparations are needed for these RNs? How many nurse educators, researchers and consultants are needed for staffing educational nursing programs and health care services, and what educational preparations are needed for these RNs?

The question of educational preparation for the various nursing positions usually provokes considerable discussion in any planning group discussing nursing requirements. This is certainly an area that needs further research investigation. The division of nursing has prepared a set of guidelines indicating criteria of educational preparation for RN positions.[10] These guidelines should be helpful as a beginning basis for negotiation in a planning group discussing the educational preparation of nurses for different types of positions.

Data Issues

Having completed the theoretical presentation of the steps in the planning process, the planner should be aware that *data* describing the current situation provides a base upon which to make decisions about the future. What then are the data that should be used to carry out the steps in the planning process? Are the data generally available? Are they reliable? How valid are they? Can they be easily understood, clearly interpreted and exposed to public scrutiny?

ANALYSIS AND PLANNING

In the Analysis and Planning Project we relied on assembling nationally available data, specific at the county level. That is, we used existing data bases acquired from a variety of agencies and organizations, which had data describing phenomena at the

There are some significant gaps in data that are needed for nursing planning. The planner concerned with nursing requirements and resources will find insufficient information about ethnicity of nurses, new and emerging nursing roles and specialties acquired by nurses.

county level. In closely reviewing these national data files, there are some significant gaps in data that are needed for nursing planning, though no more than one finds in data about other health professions. The planner concerned with nursing requirements and resources will find insufficient information about ethnicity of nurses, new and emerging nursing roles and specialties acquired by nurses. These problems are discussed and recommendations presented in detail in the project report *Long-Range Data Collection and Use.*[11]

The experience of the Analysis and Planning Project suggests that in working with state planning groups, special surveys have been conducted in which more specific and complete data exist. This is particularly true with respect to data collected by the State Department of Health. It should be noted that the National Center of Health Statistics in 1973 assumed major responsibility for developing a federal-state-local Cooperative Health Statistics System (CHSS). When this system is fully developed it is expected it will provide the necessary

136 statistical base for effective nation-wide health planning.

REVIEW OF QUESTIONS

These steps in the planning process and data issues raise a series of questions that are essential to doing state-level health planning in a credible fashion. By proceeding through the delineated process, the questions are reviewed logically and systematically so as to facilitate thorough and comprehensive health planning. The answers to the questions fit together and build upon one another so that the net result is a rational health care delivery policy that is built upon an integrated set of policy decisions. These decisions form the basis for making projections of the number and kinds of nurses who will be needed and who will be available to meet the population's health care needs. The nursing projections as well as the policy decisions which underlie the projections attempt to direct the development of the health care delivery system in a way that should be beneficial to both health care providers and the public.

We have emphasized the need for nursing administrators to be involved in extra-institutional planning and with nursing manpower issues at the state level. The real question is not whether decisions will be made at the state level which affect nursing, but whether the decisions will be made with effective nursing input.

The planning approach discussed in this article is one that provides opportunities for nursing administrators to be meaningful contributors. The issues raised in this planning process are ones that nursing administrators have had experience with in their own institutions and in which they should be able to provide leadership in planning at the state level.

REFERENCES

1. Aydelotte, M. *Nurse Staffing Methodology*. HEW Division of Nursing Pub. No. 73-433 (January 1973).
2. For a full discussion of the entire process, see Gray, R., Sauer, K. and Smith M. *Nursing Resources and Requirements: A Guide for State-Level Planning*. Division of Nursing Contract No. 321-750803 (1977) in press.
3. *Health Characteristics of Low Income Persons*. DHEW Pub. No. (HSM) 73-1500 (1972).
4. Pettigrew, A. H. and Pettigrew, T. F. "Race, Disease and Desegregation: A New Look." Shiloh A. and Selaven I., Eds. *Ethnic Groups of America: Their Morbidity, Mortality and Behavior Disorders II* (Springfield, Ill.: Charles C. Thomas (1974) p. 43–51.
5. Stamber, J. *et al.* "Racial Patterns of Coronary Heart Disease." Shiloh, A. and Selevan I., Eds.
Ethnic Groups of America: Their Morbidity, Mortality and Behavior Disorders II (Springfield, Ill.: Charles C. Thomas 1974) p. 95–98.
6. Bullough, B. and Bullough, V. L. *Poverty, Ethnic Identity and Health Care* (New York: Appleton-Century-Crofts 1972) p. 75–76.
7. Baetjer, A. "Atmospheric Pollution." Sartwell, P. E., Ed. *Maxy-Rosenau Preventive Medicine and Public Health* (10th ed.) (New York: Appleton-Century-Crofts 1973) p. 881–887.
8. Martin, J., Ed. *Comprehensive Health Planning* (Chicago: Blue Cross Association 1975).
9. Aydelotte, *Nurse Staffing Methodology*.
10. *Source Book for Nursing Personnel* DHEW Pub. No. (HRA) 75-43 (1974).
11. *Recommendations Concerning Long Range Data Collection and Use*. Division of Nursing Contract No. 321-750803, HEW (1977) in press.

NAQ Forum: Staffing

THE ROLE OF THE NURSING
ADMINISTRATOR IN STAFFING

Thelma Differt, B.S.N., *Nursing Administrator, St. Joseph's Hospital,
Milwaukee, Wisconsin:*

One can hardly address the subject of
staffing without first reviewing the road
map marked with visible landmarks that
has led you to your destination. Over the
years, as nursing administrators have
organized their departments, more
landmarks have been added to our maps.
The course has become more sophisticated and, if you will, more difficult, with
many constraints being placed upon
administrators by health care regulators.
Staffing, although it is one of the most
critical concerns facing nursing administration today, must be viewed as only one
facet of the total nursing care program.

Determining Objectives

The first landmark on your map should
reveal the philosophy and objectives of
the nursing department. The objectives
and management of nursing care
influence a staffing program and are
utilized as determinants in forecasting a

137

138 nursing budget. In developing these objectives, these issues must be addressed:

- Is your objective to provide total individual care with assessment and planned care for each individual patient by a registered nurse?
- Is your objective to utilize nursing assistants to assist with activities?
- Is your objective to provide a team approach utilizing nursing specialists and other disciplines?
- Is your philosophy predicated on patient needs?
- Does your philosophy reflect employee needs?
- Are the hospital philosophy and the nursing philosophy compatible?

Establishing Staffing Patterns

After you and your staff have agreed upon a philosophy of care and clearly defined your objectives, you will be approaching the next landmark on the route, that is, establishing staffing patterns which reflect the quality and quantity of various categories of nursing personnel to carry out the nursing care program. This is a profoundly important and difficult curve in the road. We are dealing with approximately one-fourth of hospital costs. We are also dealing with architectural designs, administrative policies, labor market, a large professional staff and, most of all, human beings—both patients and employees. Webbing all of these into a homogeneous pattern is no small task.

Staffing is the identification of nursing care needs, which is not a new concept for nursing. Florence Nightingale assessed and classified her patients according to nursing care needs by placing the most critical patients nearest the nurses' station. Those requiring less observation were placed farthest from it.

We have expanded on that concept and today we use a scaling device in which patient requirements for nursing care are expressed in quantitative terms. Staffing should represent a balance between the needs of the patient and the needs of the employee. "The lack of defined policies for staffing and outdated, time consuming methods contribute to poor utilization, poor morale and turnover."[1]

SCIENTIFIC METHODS

We can no longer play the numbers. game in determining staff. Tools utilized in the past such as nursing care hours based on census, subjective determination based on empirical evidence, nursing administrator's judgment, etc., are not sufficient today. There is a need for more scientific methods based on activities to justify staffing requests, and the nursing administrator has the responsibility of participating in such studies. Many studies have been ongoing since the fifties. However, we have seen an impetus with the trust of cost containment programs. In cooperation with our systems department at St. Joseph's, we have developed a nursing activity model which provides needed nursing care hours of appropriate levels of skills to care for patients in specific categories of dependency for each shift. This tool enables us to place our staff according to patient needs.

Today in an era of increased litigations, the nursing administrator must be cognizant of federal and state regulations relating to minimum wage, child labor, assignments and antidiscrimination. Although we may look at these as personnel functions, the nursing administrator does share equal responsibility.

BALANCING MACHINES AND PEOPLE

As we look further down the road, we see computerization of our staffing plans. Although this will add another dimension to our nursing care program and certainly a great adjunct, we cannot substitute machines for human relations which, in my opinion, is the heart of staffing. Machines will never predict human behavior, so our role will continue to be one of humanism.

Having reached the destination as planned on their maps, nursing administrators now must orchestrate nursing care programs by placing personnel in positions in which they can perform at their highest level. This way the administrator's audience can enjoy the very best care in their health care continuum. A program for growth and development for staff is essential. Nursing administrators must also advertise their acts by submitting their plans to hospital administration. "The nurse director has a responsibility to make known the degree of care patients may generally receive on the basis of the proposed plan."[2]

References

[1] Alexander, E. L., *Nursing Administration in the Hospital* (St. Louis, Missouri: C. V. Mosby Company 1972) p. 285.
[2] Di Vincent, M. *Administering Nursing Service* (Boston, Massachusetts: Little, Brown and Company 1972) p. 108.

STAFFING PERCEPTIONS: CAUSES AND CONCERNS

Julian Cicatiello, R.N., M.A., M.Ed., *Assistant Executive Director, Patient Services, Mercy Hospital, Miami, Florida:*

One of the greatest concerns of all nursing administrators throughout the United States is adequate staffing of the department of nursing service to meet the needs of the patient in conjunction with full utilization of the maximum potential of all personnel. Persistent factors that invariably affect staffing include the following: the academic qualifications and preparation of the nurses, the size, type, services and occupancy of the hospital, the acuity of illness of the patient, and the geographical location of the hospital.

Nursing in Miami

It must be understood that my comments are limited in that I refer to the nursing concerns in Miami, Florida. Geographically, Miami is considered by many as a most attractive city in which to practice nursing. However, in the Miami area proper, there are approximately 25 hospitals varying greatly in composition and size. Some of the hospitals may have a capacity of 40 beds, while others may in fact have a capacity of 1,000 beds. This area is considered to be overbedded by approximately two to three thousand beds. Having a general understanding then of this basic information regarding the structural inconsistencies among hospitals, it is obvious that fierce competiton constantly exists in an effort to recruit and retain nurses. Recruitment is not a totally insurmountable problem simply because many nurses seek to relocate in Florida initially. The dilemma occurs within a relatively short period of time, when nurses realize that Miami is not totally what they had envisioned and, in fact, does not meet their preconceived expectations. At this point, disillusionment and dissatisfaction become evident.

Ultimately, their own recourse is to return home, as they continually and

140 restlessly revert to the nurse circuit syndrome, traveling to the west coast, San Francisco, perhaps, then to Denver or once again back home, somehow never really finding their "niche."

Staffing Flexibility

Flexibility is imperative when staffing a department of nursing. In our department of nursing we realize five divisions: obstetrics, acute care, surgical specialty, psychiatry and two medical-surgical divisions. Within each of these divisions are approximately four to five units, each having about 40 beds per unit. Staffing flexibility is utilized when need becomes evident within a unit and personnel then can be relocated within the particular division to meet the need. When a nurse is hired for the acute care division, the individual is oriented in all areas. This prepares the individual for rotation, if necessary, to any of the required units and realistically assures that the nurse will function reasonably well in that setting. In fostering this concept, we provide for and promote more cohesiveness within each division.

Orientation

Our mix of professional nursing personnel is varied: 30 percent hold baccalaureate degrees, 40 percent hold associate degrees and approximately 30 percent are diploma graduates. Nurses graduating in 1977 have an excellent academic-scientific background but unfortunately lack the ability to transfer knowledge of scientific principles to the clinical setting. These graduates seem to be able to theorize the needs of the patient but are not adept at clinical performance. Practical knowledge and application of work assignments, the ability to organize and prioritize their

work and the inability to work under some uncontrollable situations are frequent inadequacies of the new graduate. In an effort to assist our nursing personnel in integration of academics and clinical applications, we have provided for an extensive orientation program. Our orientation program is mandatory for all nursing personnel.

Physician-Nurse Relationships

A common problem that appears to frustrate nurses is the physician-nurse relationship. There is a lack of understanding of the expansion of the role of nurses today, and the fact that it will continue to expand, scientifically, with sophistication and increased independence of thought and judgment. Conversely, physicians continue to strive to fulfill their role predicated on the concept of nursing 15 years ago. Nurses are trying to initiate the collegial or peer relationship in working with physicians, desiring to be part of the total team and to be recognized for their expertise in contributing specific nursing knowledge to this total team effort.

In an attempt to erradicate this misunderstanding and perpetuate modern day concepts of medicine/nursing intervention, we have established a Joint Practice Committee. This committe, comprised of physicians and nurses, attempts through periodic interfacing to share, discuss, inform and/or solve the more common and uncommon problems shared by physicians and nurses.

Changing Roles

What can the nursing administrator anticipate or realize with respect to staffing? At the present time, there are close to 1,000,000 nurses in the United

States, and they must be considered one of the largest groups of health professionals. However, with all of the manpower, we continue to be somewhat thwarted by a geographical distribution problem, which will probably never be solved. Nurses are, and will continue to be, mobile. Financially, many nurses do not need to work and are not the sole support of the household. Another reality is that many programs in nursing today are preparing nurses for more independent roles within our health settings, making the hospital appear less attractive than it was 25 years ago.

As a final consideration, commitment has been expressed by many nurse administrators to have impacted hospital staffing. It is doubtful that new staff nurses today are as committed to nursing as were their counterparts 25 years ago.

Directors of Nursing—
Satisfaction and Dissatisfaction

Christine T. Kovner, R.N., M.S.N.
Instructor
College of Nursing
Wayne State University
Detroit, Michigan

Roseann S. Oliver, R.N., M.S.N.
Health Care Consultant
Brown, Connery, Kulp, Willie, Purvell,
* Greene Law Firm*
Camden, New Jersey

DIRECTORS of nursing are responsible for providing adequate nursing care for patients in hospitals throughout the United States.[1] They also have responsibility for creating an environment conducive to implementing established nursing standards. These standards are directly related to the ultimate goal of the institution: the delivery of adequate patient care. Since directors are involved in the management, planning and coordination of patient care, their performance influences the delivery of this care, both directly and indirectly.[2]

Increasingly, for nursing directors, administrative responsibilities are replacing those for direct patient care. The literature indicates that there are increasing demands on directors to master management skills, including budgeting, finance and personnel administration.[3,4,5,6] Yet traditionally, directors of nursing have been viewed and have viewed themselves principally as expert nurse practitioners.

There are increasing demands on directors to master management skills, including budgeting, finance and personnel administration. Yet traditionally, directors of nursing have viewed themselves principally as expert nurse practitioners.

This change brings with it changes in the kinds of satisfaction and dissatisfaction nursing directors experience in their work environment. It is important that directors of nursing accept their new orientation as legitimate; perhaps when they recognize their role as legitimate they will perform it better.

THE STUDY

What factors do directors of nursing service describe as consistently leading to job satisfaction and dissatisfaction? And what is the validity of Herzberg's Motivation-Hygiene theory for the sample evaluated in this study?

Twenty-six randomly selected directors of nursing service from hospitals in an eastern urban area participated in this study. These directors had a median of 4.5 years' experience as director of nursing; the range varied from eight months to 18 years. The highest degree held was masters for 17 of the directors, baccalaureate for three and diploma for six.

Approximately one-half of the directors were asked to describe a situation in which they felt exceptionally good about their job and about half of the directors were asked to describe a situation which made them feel exceptionally bad about their job. Thought units (phrases or sentences, not necessarily direct quotes) were extracted from 25 of these descriptions (one director was unable to think of an appropriate experience) and typed on index cards by the researchers. The thought units were then analyzed and categorized individually by three independent judges who had no previous information about the directors' situations. Agreement of two of three judges constituted overall agreement.

Herzberg's Theory

Herzberg's theory describes job satisfaction and job dissatisfaction as unipolar traits rather than opposite ends of a bipolar continuum. He denotes those factors which lead to job satisfaction as motivators and those factors which lead to job dissatisfaction as hygienes. He suggests that motivators should be mentioned significantly more often in recounting satisfying job experiences and that hygienes should be mentioned significantly more often in recounting dissatisfying job experiences.[7]

Motivators were categorized in this study as follows: achievement, responsibility, recognition, work itself, advancement and possibility of growth. Hygienes were categorized as follows: hospital policy and administration, supervision-technical, interpersonal relations, working conditions, factors in personal life, job security, salary and status.

The Anchoring Scale[8]

Following a structured interview, the individual directors of nursing were asked to rank their experiences on a scale from 0–10, according to their own value systems. A rating of ten indicated the most satisfying or most dissatisfying experience they could imagine having in their nursing careers and a zero rating denoted the least satisfying or least dissatisfying experience they could imagine having in their nursing careers. The scale was used to lend some measurement of intensity to the study.

RESULTS

Achievement

The results of the study appear in Tables 1 and 2. One motivator—achievement—appeared significantly more often in situations of job satisfaction. Achievement was defined as "thoughts indicating personal accomplishment, seeing the results of one's work, successful completion of a job, solutions to problems and involvement or participation in successful change." This category also included the converse, such as failure or lack of achievement.

Achievement was mentioned in every satisfying experience recounted. These situations also elicited a strong response on the anchoring scale (scale six or higher). The directors talked about accomplishing higher standards

TABLE 1

Frequency with Which Factors Were Mentioned by Twenty-Five Directors of Nursing

Factor	Frequency of Occurrence
Work itself	50
Achievement	29
Interpersonal Relations	26
Supervision-Technical	23
Recognition	12
Hospital Policy and Administration	9
Responsibility	7
Possibility of Growth	5
Job Security	4
Working Conditions	3
Advancement	2
Salary	1
Personal Life	1
Status	0
Total Units	172

of patient care through nursing service activities, plus the growth and development of the nursing department. The directors seemed to feel that the quality of nursing in their institutions was a direct reflection of themselves.

Lack of achievement was frequently

Since the majority of directors in this study were very achievement-oriented, an implication for administrators working with these directors would be to allow them the autonomy necessary for formulating plans and goals for nursing while still providing them with the support necessary to implement those goals.

TABLE 2
Frequency with Which Factors Were Mentioned about Job Satisfaction and Job Dissatisfaction

Factor	Job Satisfaction N = 11 Stories	Job Dissatisfaction N = 14 Stories
Motivators		
Achievement	100%	64%
Recognition	82%	28%
Work Itself	72%	71%
Growth	18%	7%
Responsibility	9%	28%
Advancement	0	7%
Hygienes		
Interpersonal Relations	64%	57%
Supervision-Technical	45%	50%
Hospital Policy	9%	43%
Job Security	0	21%
Working Conditions	0	7%
Personal Life	9%	0
Status	0	0

mentioned in dissatisfying situations. These stressed items similar to those mentioned above but without successful results. Since the majority of directors in this study were very achievement-oriented, an implication for administrators working with these directors (24 were women) would be to allow them the autonomy necessary for formulating plans and goals for nursing while still providing them with the support necessary to implement those goals.

Hospital Policy

One hygiene—hospital policy—appeared significantly more often in dissatisfying situations. Hospital policy was defined as "some overall aspect of the hospital—good or bad effects of policies, adequate or inadequate management and organiza-tion." Nursing service policies were also included. The thought units mentioned in this category emphasized the directors' lack of participation in decisions on hospital planning and facilities, implying that if directors had a stronger voice in hospital policy decisions, they would perhaps not be as dissatisfied with this area. The interviews revealed a dichotomy between nursing and hospital philosophies. Incidents such as building new units without any nursing input, changes in physical facilities and inadequate staffing due to expansion are examples of problems mentioned. These directors did not feel nursing had a substantial voice in formulating hospital policy. Administrators who fail to involve the directors in projects such as these only add to the directors' dissatisfaction and may prove to be short-sighted in terms of the nursing cooperation and successful completion of a project.

Work Itself

Work itself was defined as "thoughts emanating from the actual doing of the job or the tasks of the job." This includes the opportunity to carry through an entire operation, the restriction to one minute aspect of it and descriptions of work which is routine or varied, creative, challenging or overly difficult. It also deals with work which is appropriate or inappropriate. The investigators believe that the directors are very involved in the day-to-day activities of the nursing department. They particularly appeared to be concerned with staff and staff's relationship to direct patient care.

DIRECTORS' SELF IMAGE

This category also indicated the directors' overall feeling about their jobs. This included comments related to the challenging nature of the work and frustrations regarding inadequate patient care. In spite of the directors' other responsibilities, they continued to place a high emphasis on patient care. Directors continue to see themselves as nurses rather than as managers of people.

The advantages to this self image are directly related to the patient. Directors see themselves as patients' advocates, employed to serve them and help elevate the institution's standards to care for them. This would indirectly aid the institution in providing quality health services. However, there are certain disadvantages to this philosophy, such as a problem of allegiance or loyalty. If the employing institutions do not share similar goals, directors will be torn between ideological commitment and practical considerations. Another disadvantage may be that the institution has employed directors as managers and not as patient advocates. This role conflict might be difficult for all involved. There continues to be an ambiguity in the directors' role; are they managers, expert clinicians or patient care advocates?

INTERPERSONAL RELATIONS

The investigators suggest that a large component of directors' time is involved in interpersonal relations. Analysis of this category indicated that the directors of nursing were talking about all levels of personnel, most frequently about the medical staff. This included areas such as explanation of the nursing role and acceptance as colleagues with hospital administration and the medical staff. This finding is indicative of the increasing struggle for nursing independence—a move away from the handmaiden role. It further reflects the current social trend toward female equality. One very effective means for bridging this gap is on the educational level. Interdisciplinary education, especially on the master's level, might assist directors and those they will be working with in appreciating each other's roles and responsibilities. Also, a background in interpersonal relations

148 would be helpful for directors of nursing.

Supervision-Technical

The supervision-technical hygiene was defined for this study as "the competence and fairness of the directors' superiors or the directors' willingness to delegate responsibility or to teach." The majority of dissatisfying experiences in this category mentioned a conflict situation between directors and their immediate superiors. This dealt with problems in the organizational structure such as not having direct access to administrators, but rather to the assistants or the medical directors. Since nursing is usually the largest department in the hospital, it would seem administratively advantageous to have the nursing directors report directly to the hospital administrators. This would certainly facilitate communication and allow for a better working relationship between administration and nursing service. It would also tend to involve the directors in important hospital policies and

---

Those directors who were actively involved with their supervisors and nursing staff derived satisfaction from their subordinates' personal and professional development.

---

decisions. The positive aspect of the category concerned the directors' relationships with their nursing supervisors. Those directors who were actively involved with their supervisors and nursing staff derived satisfaction from their subordinates' personal and professional development.

Money

Money was mentioned by only one director. The investigators suggest that if directors are at an income level that is adequate, a cut in salary would dissatisfy them, but a raise in salary would not remove the other factors they see as dissatisfying in their jobs.

Status

It is interesting to note that status, defined as "situations in which the respondent actually mentioned some sign of status, such as having a private office or being able to eat in the private dining room," was not mentioned at all by directors. This suggests that (1) directors have few thoughts of status or lack thereof, or (2) directors of nursing feel this is an inappropriate topic to discuss. Should the reason be the former, a private office may not influence directors' satisfaction or dissatisfaction with their jobs.

FUTURE AREAS OF INTEREST

Future research in this area should be directed to further describe what directors find satisfying and the relationship between their performance and job satisfaction.

It would also be of interest to investigate the role of directors of nursing as perceived by hospital administrators and directors of nursing. Included in this might be a comparison of the philosophies of patient care of administrators and directors of nursing.

Finally, further investigation of area of expertise needed by directors of nursing service should be compared with academic background. The guidance of such an investigation and comparison would be quite valuable to educational institutions preparing future directors of nursing and to programs geared to mid-career education.

This study, with the exception of achievement and hospital policy, did not support Herzberg's Theory. The directors of nursing in this sample mentioned motivators almost as often in satisfying situations as in dissatisfying ones. The frequency with which categories such as achievement, recognition, work itself, interpersonal relations and supervision-technical were mentioned indicates that these items are important to those who accept positions as heads of nursing departments.

REFERENCES

1. Arndt, C. and Laeger, E. "Role Strain in Diversified Role Set: the Director of Nursing Service, Part 1." *Nursing Research* XIX (May–June 1970) p. 252–253.
2. Foreman, W. "Administrators Analyze the Effectiveness of Their Directors of Nursing." *Hospital Management* (December 1969) p. 24–29.
3. Hamil, E. "The Changing Director of Nurses." *Nursing Outlook* XVII (December 1969) p. 64–65.
4. Gerard, M. "Recognizing the Nursing Service Director as an Administrator." *Hospital Progress* L (March 1969) p. 100–110.
5. Gross, M. "Should Nurses be Involved in Management." *Hospital Management* CXII (January 1969) p. 55–59.
6. Hoefflin, W. R. "The Relationship Between the Hospital Administrator and the Director of Nursing." *Hospital Forum* XIII (November 1969) p. 14, 15, 40, 41.
7. Herzberg, F., Mausner, B. and Snyderman, B. *The Motivation to Work* (New York: John Wiley and Sons 1959).
8. Kilpatrick, F. P. and Cantril, H. "Self-Anchoring Scaling: A Measure of Individual's Unique Reality Worlds." *Journal of Individual Psychology* XVI (November 1960) p. 158–173.

The Head Nurse As a Staff Nurse Satisfaction Factor

Virginia Rozell, R.N., M.S.
Research Associate
College of Nursing
University of Illinois
*   at the Medical Center*
Chicago, Illinois

IS it important to nursing service administrators to have a satisfied nursing staff? One observer described in the following way, nurses who were deprived of esteem and acceptance (major components in satisfaction): "They fail to develop potential, conform to existing patterns and level of performances or detach themselves from nursing altogether."[1] Another author stated that if nurses are not satisfied in the work setting, then conflict, frustration and feelings of failure occur that limit their contributions to nursing.[2]

ARE NURSES SATISFIED?

Head nurse-staff nurse relationships play significant roles in contributing to staff nurse satisfaction. Head nurses assume the dominant role and therefore the responsibility for the development and consequence of the relationship. The consequence, in this case, is satisfaction of staff nurses which, in

152

turn, affects the quality of patient care. Are nurses satisfied? One has only to observe the high turnover rate in nursing to determine that staff nurses are not content in their work settings.

The turnover rate of staff nurses in 1970 was reportedly 50 to 70 percent in some hospitals. It was 63 percent in Chicago hospitals.[3] The economics involved with this markedly high rate is a major concern, not to mention the effect on continuity of patient care, patient satisfaction and staff morale that accompany high turnover of

---

Based on economics alone, satisfaction of staff nurses is an issue that, when combined with the projected dire effects on patient care, assumes serious proportions.

---

nurses. The replacement cost for one staff nurse is estimated to be $1,000. If one multiplies this figure by 60 percent of the employed staff nurses in a hospital, one can anticipate the budgetary effect. Based on economics alone, satisfaction of staff nurses is an issue that, when combined with the projected dire effects on patient care, assumes serious proportions.

INFLUENCE OF HEAD NURSES

In the mid-60s head nurses were characterized as the most influential models of nursing behavior in the work setting.[4] In addition to the modeling effect, Bullock concluded in his attitudinal study that they had more autonomy within the unit than found in most organizations, and that nursing care units were, in fact, controlled by the individual head nurses rather than by institutional goals.[5,6] Under these circumstances, head nurses had the latitude of function in accord with their own perceptions, values and expectations as autonomous, influential leaders. What effect did this influential leadership have upon the satisfaction of staff nurses?

During the 50s and 60s, the relationship between immediate supervisors and workers was established as an important factor in satisfaction of the worker.[7,8] Studies of turnover and absenteeism made during this period suggest that nurses leave their positions due to discontentment with the head nurse-staff nurse relationship.[9,10] These findings are not surprising considering the profound influence attributed to this position during this period. In view of these facts, one may conclude that during the 50s and 60s head nurses were effective leaders who directly affected satisfaction of subordinates.

Declining Leadership

With regard to more recent studies in the early 70s, we find that a changing pattern has evolved. The head nurse-staff nurse relationship remains an important factor in staff nurse satisfaction.[11] However, in a study on the influence the head nurses on need satisfaction of staff nurses, the influence of head nurses was found among the least satisfied staff nurses and not found among the more satisfied nurses.[12] This suggests that staff nurses are not responding positively to head nurses as role models and they may be seeking or perhaps have found satisfactory relationships with other members of the nursing staff. If this is true, and further study would have to validate this finding, then the positive leadership of head nurses is declining. What factors contributed to this process of change within the past decade or two?

NEW DEVELOPMENTS

Since the earlier assessment of the 50s and 60s, several changes and innovations have developed in the health field that could affect the power exerted by head nurses: multiple educational levels in nursing, increase in the variety of health personnel and clinical specialization in nursing. An important sociological factor was, and is, the growing general attitude in society toward questioning or challenging persons in authority. It seems feasible that all of these factors may have been responsible for the changing leadership in the institutional setting.

DETERMINING THE INFLUENCE OF HEAD NURSES

In order to find out just what influence head nurses are having on staff nurses and how effective the leadership of head nurses is, a study was conducted using the Job Satisfaction Questionnaire developed by Porter in 1961.[13] Need satisfaction was defined, in this study, as a measure-

ment of the difference between the degree to which a need is satisfied (actual) and the degree to which an individual would like a need to be satisfied (desired) in the work setting. A typical question would be: "How much prestige is there in your position?" (actual) or "How much prestige should there be in your position?" (desired). With some modifications to suit the uniqueness of the head nurse-staff nurse relationship, Porter's questionnaire was used to try to measure satisfaction in the staff nurse position from the perceptions of both head nurses and staff nurses.

Eighty-one staff nurses and their 17 respective head nurses participated from four metropolitan area hospitals. There was great diversity among the participants in terms of the medical units in which they worked. However, criteria for the study required that the staff nurses be employed full time and the head nurses be employed for six months prior to the investigation in order that they develop a concept of the staff nurse position.

The questions were based on three hypotheses:

- Head and staff nurse perceptions of need satisfaction in the staff nures position coincide.
- Head nurse perceptions of need satisfaction and staff nurse actual satisfaction in the staff nurse position coincide.
- Head nurse perceptions of need satisfaction and staff nurse desired satisfaction in the staff nurse position coincide.

154   The degree to which the perceptions of head nurses toward staff nurses and the staff nurses toward their own positions coincide measured the degree to which head nurses were supposedly maintaining effective roles in influencing the need satisfaction of their staff nurses.

The Results

The most important result of the testing was the fact that the greater the influence of head nurses experienced by staff nurses, the less need satisfaction staff nurses felt. In fact, satisfaction of staff nurses could not be related to head nurse perceptions of satisfaction *except* in the least satisfied group. On the other hand, the greater the satisfaction of the staff nurses, the

---

Satisfaction of staff nurses is due to factors other than the influence of head nurses, and the positive leadership of head nurses seems to be declining.

---

smaller the influence of head nurses seemed to be. If this is true, satisfaction of staff nurses is due to factors other than the influence of head nurses, and the positive leadership of head nurses seems to be declining.

Staff nurses are not content, and the traditional leadership of head nurses is in the process of change. If head nurses are no longer effective leaders, in terms of positive leadership among staff nurses, then restructuring is essential in order to maintain an efficient chain of command and effec-

tive leadership within the department. These trends, or patterns of change, are not surprising considering the general movements within the health field. These trends, however, do present challenges to nursing service administrators, since they undoubtedly directly or indirectly affect patient care.

IMPACT OF HEAD NURSES' DECLINING INFLUENCE

One of the challenges is staff nurse satisfaction. In order to satisfy staff nurses, need satisfaction must be measured and opportunities must be provided within the work setting to allow staff nurses to fulfill their unmet needs. The head nurse-staff nurse relationship is one source from which staff nurses can derive satisfaction. However, since the leadership of the head nurses is in the process of change, head nurse-staff nurse relationships cannot serve as positive sources of satisfaction. This leads to the next challenge—the declining leadership of head nurses.

In considering the leadership of head nurses, the prime question is, "How effective are head nurses in meeting the needs of staff nurses?" An evaluation of the head nurse position and the individuals in the position can determine to what degree the leadership qualities of head nurses promote and maintain staff nurse satisfaction. This evaluation could identify areas of undeveloped expertise of head nurses. The in-service education department could assist in the evaluation process and, if necessary, develop classes in management, interpersonal relationships or group dynamics. On the other hand, it may be necessary to restructure the hierarchy within the department to obtain effective leadership which would result in staff nurse satifaction.

A second question related to the leadership of head nurses is, "If head nurses are not the model of nursing behavior for staff nurses, then who has assumed this influential position?" Identification of this model could be extremely valuable in defining leadership qualities that are important to staff nurses.

In this transitory period of nursing practice, evaluation and research can be effective resources in assisting

---

In this transitory period of nursing practice, evaluation and research can be effective resources in assisting nursing service administrators to make decisions that will be beneficial to nurses and patients.

---

nursing service administrators to make decisions that will be beneficial to nurses and patients.

REFERENCES

1. Reinkemeyer, M. H. "A Nursing Paradox." *Nursing Research* 17 (1968) p. 4–8.
2. Benton, D. A. and White, H. C. "Satisfaction of Job Factors for Registered Nurses." *Journal of Nursing Administration* 2 (1972) p. 55–63.
3. National Commission on Nursing and Nursing Education. *An Abstract for Action* (New York: McGraw-Hill Book Co. 1970).
4. Smith, K. M. "Discrepancies in the Role Specific Values of Head Nurses and Nursing Educators." *Nursing Research* 14 (1965) p. 196–202.
5. Bullock, R. P. *What Do Nurses Think of Their Profession?* (Columbus, Ohio: The Ohio State University Research Foundation 1954).
6. Grivest, M. T. "Personal Inventory of Supervisors, Head Nurses and Staff Nurses in Selected Hospitals." *Nursing Research* 7 (1958) p. 77–87.
7. Bullock, R. P. "Position, Function and Job Satisfaction of Nurses in the Social System of a Modern Hospital." *Nursing Research* 2 (1953) p. 4–14.
8. Herzberg, F., Mausner, B., Peterson, R. O. and Capwell, D. *Job Attitudes: Review of Research and Opinion* (Pittsburgh: Psychological Service of Pittsburgh 1957).
9. Diamond, L. K. and Fox, D. J. "Turnover Among Hospital Student Nurses." *Nursing Outlook* 6 (1958) p. 388–391.
10. Seleh, S. D., Lee, R. J. and Prien, E. P. "Why Nurses Leave Their Jobs—An Analysis of Female Turnover." *Personnel Administration* 27 (1965) p. 25–28.
11. Longest, B. B. "Job Satisfaction for Registered Nurses in the Hospital Setting." *Journal of Nursing Administration* 4 (1974) p. 46–52.
12. Rozell, V. L. *Need Satisfaction: A Study of the Degree of Congruence in Perceptions Between Staff Nurses and Their Head Nurses on Satisfaction of Needs Within the Position of Staff Nurse* (University of Illinois Medical Center 1976).
13. *Ibid.*

Nurse Staffing After Hospitals Merge

Elsie Ann Schmied, R.N., B.G.S., M.M.
Director of Methods Improvement for
  Nursing
Northwestern Memorial Hospital
Chicago, Illinois

"We need more nurses!" complained the physicians. "We're too short-staffed to give adequate patient care!" cried the nurses. "The nurse staffing budget is too high!" pronounced the budget manager. It was in this setting that I got involved in nurse staffing statistics.

In the world of pure research, one can set limits on a problem. Researchers look at the effect of a few variables on a situation and come up with a neat package of data. In my world, things aren't as "neat." In 1974, the director of nursing service assigned me to look at staffing and to come up with data to formulate staffing practices. This doesn't sound too complicated until you look at the situation. This study of staffing practices took place in an everchanging environment in which practices, task assignments, responsibilities and attitudes were fluctuating.

PROBLEM

The hospital was the result of a recent consolidation of two hospitals which were similar in services but different in other aspects. One had the traditional supervisor/head nurse line relationships and had begun decentralization of staffing responsibility; the other had central staffing, large supervisory spans of control and no head nurses. One had a formal differentiation of surgical patients by sex (male floors, female floors); in the other, most patients were located by service (orthopedics, ENT, etc.). The effect of this second difference was that nurses were more flexible in moving from one unit to another in the former situation; the staffing policies in the other building required nurses to float, but RNs were less flexible because of their specialization.

Nurse staffing at one hospital was considered "good" before the consolidation; during two of the previous three years, all budgeted positions were filled, at least part of the year; the other had had an acute shortage of nurses. Because of the shortage of professional nursing personnel, large numbers of LPNs and nursing

During the past five years, the nursing profession has been changing. The thrust is toward greater RN involvement in patient care and patient teaching by all levels of RNs, including the head nurse and supervisor.

assistants were used to deliver care. The RNs spent much of their time giving medications and treatments, checking orders and charting.

During the past five years, the nursing profession has been changing. The thrust is toward greater RN involvement in patient care and patient teaching by all levels of RNs, including both levels of middle management— the head nurse and supervisor. Job satisfaction increases in direct proportion to this involvement.

When the director of nursing instituted smaller spans of control for supervisors and decentralized some of the decision making, staffing and morale had improved.

GOALS

Assuming that an intensified recruitment drive would secure more RNs, three goals were set:

1. Utilize the professional nurse as fully as possible in performing only nursing functions.
2. Reorganize the structure of the nursing service department to increase the proportion of personnel giving direct patient care.
3. Decentralize authority to return the RN to the bedside, planning and giving the care or directly supervising it. This would be facilitated by having a clinical supervisor assigned to each floor

and a head nurse in charge of each discrete unit.

The director of nursing had faced a similar situation when she first came to the smaller hospital. When she instituted smaller spans of control for supervisors and decentralized some of the decision making, staffing and morale had improved. Therefore, she decided to do the same for the newly consolidated department. Change came slowly; there was much opposition at first. It took over a year of patient persuasion and many meetings to reorganize, assess and promote candidates, and to begin their development into managers.

To implement the plan, budgeted positions had to be secured. The first fiscal year we negotiated with the manager of the budget, changing LPN positions to supervisor and head nurse positions; some other non-professional positions were converted to staff nurse positions.

PATIENT CLASSIFICATION

The fiscal affairs officer presented a proposal for nurse staffing and scheduling by patient classification. We went through the literature and agreed that enough data were available so we would not have to take the industrial engineering approach. Aydelotte's review was most helpful.[1] Instead, we agreed to follow a four-class system, patterned after JCAH guidelines.[2] As a baseline, we agreed to use historical data. The number of hours per patient day was derived by taking the previous year's number of

patient days divided by the number of paid nursing hours; the quotient was 4.2. Since nursing and fiscal affairs both wanted to increase patient care hours, we mutually set 4.3 as our base. Further, we agreed to use this standard only for medical and surgical floors; obstetrics, psychiatry and intensive care units would be addressed later.

Table 1 is our working agreement: patient care classification according to nursing care requirements. The most valuable feature of this categorization procedure is that it provides for more help when there is a genuine increase in highly demanding patients. Similarly, it indicates where and how much staff can be reduced when the inevitable swing back to less acute conditions occurs. Head nurses become secure in knowing that their units are staffed according to need, rather than simple bed occupancy; the cycle of feast or famine is broken.

Table 2 illustrates the broad criteria developed for classifying patients based upon dependency needs, *not* task orientation.

Once the staff was familiar with the system, daily patient classification by the head nurse started on all medical and surgical floors. Each month, I manually averaged seven consecutive days of data for each unit. Within six months I had enough data to prepare a staffing budget for every unit, based upon patient needs; additional RN positions were justified and approved.

The manual system was too cumbersome to use for daily staffing without added involvement, so we

TABLE 1
Patient Classification According to Nursing Care Requirements

1. OBJECTIVES
   - Provide the required number of hours for appropriate care of the total patient load.
   - Be predictive: The staffing of a unit should be based on the number of kinds of patients actually to be found there when the shift begins.
   - Allocate staff flexibility according to patient load, the actual nursing care required by those patients, the relative amounts of care provided per shift, and the varying needs of each unit.
   - Incorporate within itself the management controls necessary to maintain an accepted performance standard.

2. STANDARDS FOR SCHEDULING
   Set standard hours per patient day for each nursing unit, at 287,000 patient days*, by two major categories: professional and non-professional.

   - Professional staff are RNs, including head nurses.
   - Non-professional staff include LPNs, aides, technicians and unit secretaries.

   - Pro-rate 51% for the day shift
       34% for the evening shift
       15% for the night shift

   - Standard = 4.3 manhours per patient day

Professional	= 1.9	44%
Non-Professional	= 2.4	56%
	4.3	100%

3. STANDARDS FOR CLASSIFYING PATIENTS

Category	Description	Relate to Standard Hours
I	Minimum Care	65% of Standard Hours
II	Average Care	100% of Standard Hours
III	Above Average Care	135% of Standard Hours
IV	Maximum Care	200% of Standard Hours

4. SCHEDULING OF STAFF
   - Establish "permanent" nursing staff by unit at a number sufficient to service an occupancy level of approximately 70 percent. "Rotating" or "relief" staff is calculated, making up the difference to standard hours calculated in Number 2.
   - Establish a format whereby the prediction of the number of patients by category and required nursing hours for the *oncoming* shift should be done by the head nurse of the present shift, so that in effect, the head nurses are never involved in planning staff for their own shifts, but instead, do it for each other.

*Projected patient days for that year.

TABLE 2
Criteria for Classification According to Nursing Care Requirements

I. (65%) A PATIENT WHO REQUIRES ONLY MINIMAL AMOUNT OF NURSING CARE

(An average of 2.8 nursing hours per 24 hours)

Examples

- A patient who is mildly ill (generally termed convalescent).
- A patient who requires little treatment and/or observation and/or instruction.
- A patient who is up and about as desired; takes his own bath or shower.
- A patient who does not exhibit any unusual behavior patterns.
- A patient without intravenous therapy or many medications.

II. (100%) A PATIENT WHO REQUIRES AN AVERAGE AMOUNT OF NURSING CARE

(An average of 4.3 nursing hours per 24 hours)

Examples

- A patient whose extreme symptoms have subsided or not yet appeared.
- A patient who requires periodic treatments and/or observations and/or instructions.
- A patient who is up and about with help for limited periods; partial bed rest required.
- A patient who exhibits some psychological or social problems.
- A patient with intravenous therapy with medications such as IV piggybacks every six hours.
- A newly admitted patient, either surgical or medical, who is a routine admission and not necessarily acutely ill.

III. (135%) A PATIENT WHO REQUIRES ABOVE AVERAGE NURSING CARE

(An average of 5.8 nursing hours per 24 hours)

Examples

- A moderately ill patient.
- A patient who requires treatments or observations as frequently as every two to four hours.
- A patient with significant changes in treatment or medication orders more than four times a day.
- An uncomplicated patient with IV medications every four hours and/or hyperalimentation.
- A patient on complete bed rest.

IV. (200%) A PATIENT WHO REQUIRES MAXIMUM NURSING CARE

(An average of 8.6 nursing hours per 24 hours)

This classification is most often used in intensive care areas.

Examples

- A patient who exhibits extreme symptoms (usually termed acutely ill).
- A patient whose activity must be rigidly controlled.
- A patient who requires continuous treatment and/or observations and/or instructions.
- A patient with significant changes in doctor's orders, more than six times a day.
- A patient with many medications, IV piggybacks, and vital signs every hour and/or hourly output.

The total amount of time required to care for each patient determines his classification.

162 continued data collection for another year. It was invaluable when we opened a new wing.

COMPUTERIZATION

By 1976, I was able to get a simple computer program written and run so that we could predict staffing needs on a daily basis. Table 3 is a sample prediction for one building. The environment also changed; to compare actual with projected staffing, we had actual staffing added to the program. For the first few months there were numerous errors to correct, but the data did support the department's assertion that as the length of stay decreased, the intensity of care required increased: a greater number of category-four patients and a decrease in category-one patients. However, as soon as there were major discrepancies (in

The data did support the department's assertion that as the length of stay decreased, the intensity of care required increased.

either direction) between actual and projected staffing, some head nurses set a low priority on patient classification, and data were either late or missing.

By fall of 1976, the data were still used only for budgeting. When ten units were moved to consolidate services geographically, it was the only reasonable basis for assessing the budgetary needs of each unit. Using the data, the only variable was the comparative number of beds. For example, when the ENT service went from 24 to 30 beds, the staffing budget was adjusted accordingly.

TABLE 3
Sample Computer Printout

04/23/77			HOSPITAL					PAGE NO 2	
10			DAILY PROJECTED STAFFING						
	HOSP	2ND SHIFT		3RD SHIFT		1ST SHIFT		PROJ DAYS TOTAL	
WING	CODE	R.N.	NONPROF.	R.N.	NONPROF.	R.N.	NONPROF.	R.N.	NONPROF.
4 WEST	2	2.63	2.86	1.16	1.26	3.95	4.29	7.74	8.41
5 EAST	2	3.39	3.53	1.50	1.56	5.08	5.29	9.97	10.37
5 WEST	2	1.53	1.59	.68	.70	2.30	2.39	4.50	4.68
6 EAST	2	3.08	3.89	1.36	1.72	4.63	5.83	9.07	11.43
6 WEST	2	1.87	2.36	.83	1.04	2.81	3.55	5.51	6.95
7 EAST	2	1.49	1.87	.66	.82	2.23	2.80	4.38	5.49
7 WEST	2	.67	.84	.29	.37	1.00	1.25	1.96	2.46
8 EAST	2	1.59	2.00	.70	.88	2.38	2.99	4.67	5.87
8 WEST	2	.94	1.19	.42	.52	1.42	1.78	2.77	3.49
9 EAST	2	2.05	2.58	.91	1.14	3.08	3.87	6.03	7.59
		19.24	22.71	8.51	10.01	28.88	34.04	56.60	66.74

PRESENT STATUS

Now that the units are all specialized, it is not feasible to use the scheduling system in Table 1. The possibility of using "floats" decreased as the degree of specialization of the units increased. Head nurses are responsible for staffing their units, and moving staff is only practical within a specialty; medicine and other specialties with more than one unit have that flexibility.

The real world presented us with complex problems. I was able to devise a practical method to use; now that it is programmed into the computer, ratios of RNs to nonprofessionals and proportions of staff on the various shifts can easily be

---

The real world presented us with complex problems . . . now that it is programmed into the computer, ratios of RNs to nonprofessionals and proportions of staff on the various shifts can easily be changed.

---

changed. The system functions, but needs refining. Until the users are committed to using data by which to staff, it has only limited value.

THE FUTURE

Where can we go from here? The road has a number of forks:
- We can build into the program the qualifications needed; not just "RN" but "BSN RN", "AD RN" and the like.
- With a good data base and a slightly more involved program, a computerized scheduling system can evolve.
- Patient room rates could be adjusted according to care received.[3]

Staffing according to patient care needs is relatively new. We've always given help to busy units. This system is one way to quantify how busy a unit is and what kind of help to send. To paraphrase Neil Armstrong when he stepped out on the moon, it's one giant step for patient care staffing.

REFERENCES

1. Aydelotte, M. *Nurse Staffing Methodology—A Review and Critique of Selected Literature* (Washington, D.C., HEW Pub. No. (NIH)73-433 1973).
2. Joint Commission on Accreditation of Hospitals. *Nursing Services* (Chicago: Joint Commission on Accreditation of Hospitals 1973) p. 6.
3. Wood, C. and Goldman, M. "Interrelated Programs in Split-Cost Accounting, Prescheduling and Peer Review." *Proceedings of the Fifth Annual Conference of the Hospital Management Systems Society* (February 1977) p. 210–231.

Patient Care Needs—An Index for Community Health Staffing

Gretchen Regnery, M.S.N., R.N.
Senior Field Supervisor
Visiting Nurse Association of Milwaukee
Milwaukee, Wisconsin

The problem of staffing the health care agency is one of the most complex and perplexing problems with which nursing administrators have to cope. For cost effectiveness and work efficiency, it is essential to utilize the available personnel well. It is also extremely important to document the need for additional personnel.

STAFFING STUDIES

Stevens claims that "... in determining staffing needs, most nurse executives use a combination of tradition, staff feedback and staffing theory. This mixture may be generously laced with trial and error."[1] That such a haphazard approach to staffing is still being used by some nurse administrators is amazing considering the wealth of information on staffing methodologies found in the literature.

Aydelotte describes four major staffing methodologies—descriptive,

166   industrial engineering, management engineering and operations research.[2] These methodologies indicate a gradual sophistication and growing attempt to gather data that are more reliable and more pertinent. Several problems arise in each of the four methodologies because they include subjective judgment, lack of quality care or quality performance measurements, lack of testing for accuracy in reporting and in training observers, and use of face validity.[3] No one report or study has attempted to deal with the entire complex of components relative to staffing because such a task would be monumental. Most studies have dealt with *one* aspect or tested *one* methodology.

The problem of staffing the community health agency has received less attention in the literature. Several unique problems arise when discussing the staffing for community health services. Roberts summarizes several of these unique features as follows:

> Since public health, in its broadest sense, is but one part of the social structure interdependent with the educational, economic, political and historical pattern of the community, each aspect of public health is in turn strongly influenced by each of the other integral parts. Thus, the staffing of [public] health services is firmly rooted in the matrix of the society served. . . .[4]

> Undoubtedly, the most important single requisite of the staffing plan is that it be designed locally, tailored to the specifications of the individual community. This implies a continuous process of evaluation, planning and demonstration of services. . . .[5]

Roberts proposes a combination of the descriptive approach and the work sampling method to determine staffing requirements. Her approach is twofold—estimating the type and amount of service to be provided and translating this estimate into personnel required to provide the service. To accomplish this process, the following information must be collected: "(1) determination of services provided per year, (2) enumeration of service requirements, and (3) staff required for intended service."[6] The information is then translated into mathematical computations. For example, the formula for estimating time available for nursing service in one year equals the staff available for service multiplied by the working days per nurse per year.

Counting Methods

Traditionally, community health nursing administrators have used one or more "counting" methods for determining staffing patterns. These may consist of determining the total population of geographical area, or concentrating on a particular age group in that area and dividing this number among the nursing staff available. Both these counting methods assume that the health care needs of the population chosen are identical despite differences in the distribution of age groups, sex, race and socioeconomic factors. They also assume that all community health nurses are equally competent.

In the same way, the number of referrals from hospitals, schools and

> *Counting activities or tasks uses an industrial engineering approach to staffing. The number of direct and indirect nursing tasks are correlated to the amount of time being spent in those tasks.*

private physicians are distributed among the nursing staff in another counting method. However, no provision is made to evaluate the *need* for the referral or the complexity of the problem.

Counting activities or tasks uses an industrial engineering approach to staffing. The number of direct and indirect nursing tasks are correlated to the amount of time being spent in those tasks. Yet answers are sought to questions such as the following from a Kissinger study: "Given the nursing staff available, are all nurses fulfilling their roles to optimum capacity? Can they extend themselves further? Are there tasks which could be done by individuals with less training?"[7] Although counting methods determine the amount of time spent on each activity, they are quantitative approaches and require interpretation of data.

Patient Care Classification Methods

Counting method approaches to staffing do not consider the degree of nursing care needed. Some attempts to overcome this shortcoming were made by Georgette and Pardee through patient classification to determine nursing needs. Both claim

that patient classification systems will lead to better staffing patterns. Georgette conducted a study of patient classification that included activities such as ". . . extensive patient teaching, reassuring the apprehensive patient, and the demanding patient who frequently takes a great deal of time."[8] Pardee developed a three-category system that classified patients according to the amount of care needed, from minimal to total, and used the most common conditions, procedures and treatments, as criteria for classification.[9]

The purpose of both of these studies was to adjust staffing by determining the number of patients needing certain levels of care. While this purpose was fine in theory, it was highly subjective, and bias and error of each nurse was not taken into consideration. Also, they did not describe how much agreement there was in the classification of the same patient by two or more nurses. Yet even with these disadvantages, the patient care classification system developed in the Georgette and Pardee studies was a breakthrough for nursing in developing a staffing methodology.

One example of a patient care classification system for community health nursing is reported by Price.[10] In this method, patients are placed into one of three categories—essential nursing care, progressive nursing care or comprehensive nursing care. Specific criteria are described for each category and a specific level of personnel is assigned for each category.

Taking a different approach to the

classification problem, Tapia developed ". . . a model for family nursing based on a continuum of five levels of family functioning."[11] The model was developed by studying the tasks of the nuclear family, namely, to provide for security and physical survival, emotional and social functioning, sexual differentiation and training of children and growth of individual members, plus the family's ability to accomplish these tasks.[12] Tapia states that the family's level of functioning or coping is an indication of its health state so that any change in that functioning level also indicates a change in its health status.[13]

Family Coping Index

The Johns Hopkins School of Public Health and the Richmond Instructive Visiting Nurses Association developed a Family Coping Index.[14] "The purpose of the Family Coping Index is to provide a basis for estimating the nursing needs of a particular family."[15] Several basic assumptions regarding the nursing process were made when developing this tool, including: (1) nursing care or intervention will make a difference in a family's ability to cope with their health problems; (2) nursing care needs can be defined in nursing terms and are based on the health problem itself, the attitudes and knowledge of the family, the availability of medical and hospital resources plus other social and environmental factors; and (5) diagnosis of nursing needs in terms of nursing intervention required should help the nurse to orga-

> *In using the Family Coping Index, the nurse assesses the family's ability to cope within nine broad categories encompassing physical independence, therapeutic competence, knowledge of health conditions, application of principles of general hygiene, etc.*

nize and plan nursing care with precision thereby inhibiting ritualistic responses. In using the Family Coping Index, the nurse assesses the family's ability to cope within nine broad categories encompassing physical independence, therapeutic competence, knowledge of health conditions, application of principles of general hygiene, health attitudes, emotional competence, family living, physical environment and use of community resources.

While these studies do not purport to be classification systems, many of the ideas and concepts identified and discussed could be incorporated in the development of such a system for use in community health. The methodology used for patient care classification in community health must be structured to consider the patient's and/or family's priorities for nursing/health care.

A PROJECT TO SOLVE STAFFING PROBLEMS

The nursing administrator of one metropolitan area community health agency found the staffing pattern there to be inadequate. It neither documented the need for additional personnel nor did it effectively utilize the available personnel (some personnel were overworked whereas others were seeking "something to do"). A project was initiated in an attempt to deal with these problems through the development and testing of a patient care classification tool to later be implemented if successfully tested.

The project was divided into three phases: (1) the development of the patient care classification tool; (2) testing the tool for validity/reliability; and (3) analyzing the data.

The development of the tool itself resulted in a four-level classification instrument. From the work of Rivers, the concepts of intensive supervision, periodic supervision and limited supervision were adapted to develop the broad definitions for each of the care levels. Price's categories of comprehensive nursing care, essential nursing care and progressive nursing care were also used in developing the care level definitions. Subcategories, developed using concepts from Tapia, Roberts, Georgette and the Richmond Instructive Visiting Nurses Association, included: family, situation, physical independence, therapeutic competence, knowledge of health conditions, health attitudes, applications of principles of general hygiene, physical environment, community resources, emotional/behavioral and public health priorities. The subcategories each had several descriptive criteria. Each subcategory was found in all four levels with the criteria characterizing the subcategory being appropriate to the care level in which it was placed.

Testing

To test the tool, the case summary of ten patients, randomly chosen, and a copy of the patient care classification tool developed in Phase I of the project were distributed to the nursing administrative personnel. The nurses were instructed to read the case summaries and to place or classify the patients into the care level which was most appropriate to their condition. The individual nurses were asked to use their expertise to select the definitions that they believed fit each level and the criteria that they believed fit each subcategory within that level. The results were tabulated and compared.

Several interesting items were discovered as a result of the tabulations and comparisons. The broad definitions for Level I and Level II were agreed upon by all four experts (100 percent). The definitions for Level III and Level IV were agreed upon by three experts (75 percent) but were reversed by the fourth expert. Since the fourth expert defined Level III the way the other experts defined Level IV, Level III was considered as Level IV and Level IV as Level III when comparing the criteria. In order for a criterion to be considered valid, it had to be agreed upon by three out of the four experts. The three experts had to agree to both the care level into which it was placed and to the subcategory

TABLE 1
Patient Care Classification
LEVEL I

DEFINITION: This category of care includes those patients and/or families requiring intensive public health nursing service. This category comprises patients who demand a high degree of nursing skill in utilizing knowledge of the physical and behavioral sciences, in in-depth analysis of the patient's needs and problems, in formulation of the nursing care plan and in therapeutic treatment of the patient and family.

Family Situation	Psychological Component	Therapeutic Competence	Knowledge of Health Conditions	Health Attitudes	Principles of General Hygiene	Environmental Milieu	Community Resources
This category includes criteria which broadly describe the family and how it is coping as a unit with its developmental tasks.	This category includes criteria relating to the emotional health of the family as a whole and/or of the individual members.	This category includes criteria pertaining to treatments, procedures and medications prescribed for the care of illness.	This category includes criteria relating to the acquisition of information about the particular health condition that is the occasion for care.	This category includes criteria which describe the way the family feels about health care in general.	This category includes criteria which describe activities of daily living such as personal care, personal hygiene, nutrition, sleep and relaxation and which relate to completing needed immunizations.	This category includes criteria concerned with the condition of the house and the type of neighborhood in which the patient/family lives.	This category includes criteria which describe the degree to which the family knows about and uses area agencies and facilities
Disorganization in all areas of family life.	Family/patient have deep-seated emotional or behavioral problems or such problems are suspected.	Family/patient either not carrying out procedures or treatments or are not doing it safely.	Family/patient totally uninformed about health condition or health problem.	Family/patient resents or resists all health care providers	Necessary immunizations not secured for children and/or adults.	House in poor condition—lead or safety hazards exist.	No community activities exist or are participated in; family/patient has no hobbies or outside interests.
Family does not meet its needs for security and physical survival.	One or more family member's reactions to illness, disability and stress need professional intervention.	Family/patient not giving or taking medications as prescribed.	Family/patient has lack of knowledge about the disease or disability as it relates to cause and effect.		Family members unkempt, dirty, inadequately clothed; diet grossly inadequate or unbalanced; children and adults getting too little sleep.	Overcrowding exists.	Family/patient unaware of and unwilling to utilize community resources.
Family has inability to secure adequate wages or to budget money.	Family/patient does not recognize their obvious and serious health and/or social needs or problems.	Family/patient fail to keep scheduled medical appointments and/or appointments with other professional services (P.T., O.T., social services) as prescribed.			Family fails entirely in providing required personal care to one or more of its members.	Neighborhood deteriorated.	
Members of family not working; dependent on public assistance or fixed income.	Family/patient does not face reality.					Community environment is totally unsatisfactory or unsafe; alcoholism or drug abuse problems suspected or known.	
Family expresses alienation from the community—lack of trust of outsiders, hostile, resistant.						Rodent or insect problem known or suspected.	

TABLE 2
Patient Care Classification
LEVEL II

DEFINITION: This category of care includes those patients and/or families requiring regular public health nursing service. This category comprises patients who need nursing care to achieve a higher level of independence and who need continuous evaluation of their health status.

Family Situation	Psychological Component	Therapeutic Competence	Knowledge of Health Conditions	Health Attitudes	Principles of General Hygiene	Environmental Milieu	Community Resources
This category includes criteria which broadly describe the family and how it is coping as a unit with its developmental tasks.	This category includes criteria relating to the emotional health and social functioning of the family as a whole and/or of the individual members.	This category includes criteria pertaining to treatments, procedures and medications prescribed for the care of illness.	This category includes criteria relating to the acquisition of information about the particular health condition that is the occasion for care.	This category includes criteria which describe the way the family feels about health care in general.	This category includes criteria which describe activities of daily living such as personal care, personal hygiene, nutrition, sleep and relaxation and which relate to completing needed immunizations.	This category includes criteria concerned with the condition of the house and the type of neighborhood in which the family/patient lives.	This category includes criteria which describe the degree to which family knows about and uses area agencies and facilities.
Family life may be less disorganized in many areas.	Family must struggle to provide for emotional health and social functioning of family members.	Family/patient is carrying out some but not all of the prescribed procedures or treatments; PHN support and encouragement required.	Family/patient has the information concerning the health condition or health problem but actions do not indicate that the information is being applied in the situation.	Family/patient accept health care only in crisis situations or in care of serious illness/no preventive health care is sought.	Some initial immunizations secured but follow-up immunizations not pursued.	House in fair condition—safety hazards exist but family could rectify if identified.	Few community activities to participate in; family/patient has few hobbies or outside interests.
Family barely meets its needs for security and physical survival.	One or more family members expresses anxiety, guilt, depression or inability to cope with stress.	Family/patient giving or taking medications correctly but does not understand purposes of the drug or symptoms to be observed.	Family/patient has some general knowledge of the disease or condition but fails to grasp the underlying principles or is only partially informed.		Family/patient generally meeting hygiene needs of sleep, nutrition and cleanliness but need reinforcement, reminders and on-going teaching and help with these measures.	Overcrowding exists but house livable.	Family/patient know some community resources but no help to use appropriate resources.
Family finances are able to meet expenses of daily living but cannot meet any type of crisis.	Family/patient usually recognizes their obvious health or social problems or needs but need help in identifying the less obvious needs or problems.	Family/patient not consistently following through with scheduled medical appointments and/or appointments with other professional services or only following through with PHN assistance or effort.			Family is providing partially for personal care needs of its members or is providing personal care for some members but not for others.	Neighborhood poor.	
Members of family are forced to work beyond reasonable limits (household head holding two or more jobs).						Some juvenile or adult delinquency among neighbors known or suspected.	
Although still alienated from the community, some beginning trust is evident in the family.							

TABLE 3
Patient Care Classification
LEVEL III

DEFINITION: This category of care includes those patients and/or families requiring occasional public health nursing service. This category comprises patients who require nursing care for therapeutic purposes and for being maintained in their homes or to avoid institutionalization.

Family Situation	Psychological Component	Therapeutic Competence	Knowledge of Health Conditions	Health Attitudes	Principles of General Hygiene	Environmental Milieu	Community Resources
This category includes criteria which broadly describe the family and how it is coping as a unit with its developmental tasks.	This category includes criteria relating to the emotional health of the family as a whole and/or of the individual members.	This category includes criteria pertaining to treatments, procedures and medications prescribed for the care of illness.	This category includes criteria relating to the acquisition of information about the particular health condition that is the occasion for care.	This category includes criteria which describe the way the family feels about health care in general.	This category includes criteria which describe activities of daily living such as personal care, personal hygiene, nutrition, sleep and relaxation and which relate to completing needed immunizations.	This category includes criteria concerned with the condition of the house and the type of neighborhood in which the family/patient lives.	This category includes criteria which describe degree to which family knows about and uses area agencies and facilities.
Family situation is essentially normal but it has more than a healthy amount of conflicts and problems.	Family/patient has reached its highest level of functioning within its resources and environment but may need PHN intervention to keep from deteriorating.	Family/patient demonstrates ability to carry out procedures and treatments; may need some PHN support and encouragement to continue.	Generally family/patient knows and accepts health condition or problem but may need PHN teaching support and supervision to avoid lapses into old patterns.	Family/patient may understand and recognize need for medical care in illness.	Immunizations generally complete for children and adults.	House in good repair but safety hazards may be present that need PHN evaluation.	Community activities provided but access may present some problems; family/patient has some hobbies and outside interests but need encouragement to continue participation.
Members are beginning to meet their need for security and physical survival.	One or more family members may be lacking in emotional control.	Family/patient giving or taking medications as prescribed with fairly good understanding of the purposes for and symptoms to be observed but needs some PHN supervision.			Family/patient able to apply most general principles of hygiene.	Overcrowding not a problem although living space may be small and cramped.	Family/patient knows and uses community resources but may need PHN intervention to continue to follow through.
Family finances are adequate for most situations except long-term or disastrous types of conditions.	Family/patient recognizes problems but their problem-solving approach needs improvement.	Family/patient following through with scheduled medical appointments and/or appointments with other professional services but may need PHN reminders and encouragement.			Family providing for personal care needs of its members but only with PHN encouragement and support.	Neighborhood borderline to respectable.	
Members of family working above normal limits.						Some undesirable social elements exist but able to protect children from poor social influences.	
Family demonstrates a greater trust in people and in the community; limited alienation may persist.							

172

TABLE 4
Patient Care Classification
LEVEL IV

DEFINITION: This category of care includes those patients and/or families requiring limited public health nursing service. This category comprises patients who require nursing care in times of crisis or on a short-term basis for resolving health problems or for referral to other agencies.

Family Situation	Psychological Component	Therapeutic Competence	Knowledge of Health Conditions	Health Attitudes	Principles of General Hygiene	Environmental Milieu	Community Resources
This category includes criteria which broadly describe the family and how it is coping as a unit with its developmental tasks.	This category includes criteria relating to the emotional health of the family as a whole and/or of the individual members.	This category includes criteria pertaining to treatments, procedures and medications prescribed for the care of illness.	This category includes criteria relating to the acquisition of information about the particular health condition that is the occasion for care.	This category includes criteria which describe the way the family feels about health care in general.	This category includes criteria which describe activities of daily living such as personal care, personal hygiene, nutrition, sleep and relaxation and which relate to completing needed immunizations.	This category includes criteria concerned with the condition of the house and the type of neighborhood in which the family/patient lives.	This category includes criteria which describe the degree to which family knows about and uses area agencies and facilities.
Family is normal, stable and healthy with a fewer than usual number of problems which they are normally able to handle as they arise.	Crisis may immobilize the family but they have the ability to adapt and change, enjoy the present and plan for the future.	Family/patient is able to demonstrate that they can carry out the prescribed procedures safely and effectively with an understanding of the principles involved and with a confident, willing attitude.	Family/patient know salient facts about the disease or problem well enough to take necessary action at the proper time.	Family/patient understands, recognizes and accepts the need for health care.	Immunizations complete for all children and adults according to standard recommendations.	House in good repair—no safety hazards identifiable.	Many opportunities for community activities; family/patient has hobbies and outside interests which they enjoy.
The family's physical survival and security needs are met.	All family members are able to maintain a reasonable degree of emotional calm.	Family/patient giving or taking medications as prescribed and knows purposes for and symptoms to be observed with each.	Family/patient understand the rationale of care and are able to observe and report significant symptoms.		Personal hygiene excellent; family meals well selected and well balanced; habits of sleep and rest adequate to needs.	No crowding exists adequate living space is present providing for privacy of all family members.	Family/patient use available resources and suitable facilities as needed.
Family finances are usually not a problem.	Family/patient recognizes its problems and develops solutions.	Family/patient giving or taking medications as prescribed and knows purposes for and symptoms to be observed with each.			All family members, whether or not there is infirmity or disability in one or more of its members, are receiving the necessary personal care.	Neighborhood respectable.	
Members of family working at a normal limit (household head is not working more than one job).	The family faces reality realistically and optimistically.	Family/patient following through with medical appointments and with appointments with other professionals.				Neighborhood free from undesirable social elements.	
No alienation exists.						Home is free of rodent and pest problems.	

174 into which it fit. If such agreement was not present, the criterion was discarded. Tables 1 through 4 display the finalized patient care classification tool.

The final test of the tool involved 25 patient charts. Each participant was requested to place each of the 25 patients into a patient care level using the information contained in the case summary and by applying the definitions of the care levels and the subcategories with their criteria.

Using the data of the 25 participants in the study, the overall reliability coefficient was approximately .84, which was above the expected .75. The tool was tested through research design and was felt to be valid and reliable for use within the agency.

Recommendations

An evaluation by the agency of the classification tool they had developed and implemented resulted in the following recommendations:

- Each criterion within the tool should be more specifically defined. This procedure could include a creation of a range of possible situations for each care level into which the criterion might fit.
- It might be possible to determine if it is correct to assume that when the nursing or patient/family problem is complex, more nursing time is required to solve the problem or vice versa.
- The patient care classification system might be used in several

If applicable, this patient classification methodology for utilization and assignment of community health nurses would provide valuable data for budgetary concerns relating to manpower requirements needed for a specific community's health service.

situations—as an overall profile of community health nurses' caseloads on a daily, weekly or monthly basis; as an overall profile of nurses' caseloads at the time of caseload reviews; or as a profile of the patient/family by scoring the patient/family on each of the subcategories thereby permitting measurement of progress if the scoring is again completed after a certain period of nursing intervention.

- The system should be tested in several other community health agencies. If applicable, this methodology for utilization and assignment of community health nurses would provide valuable data for budgetary concerns relating to manpower requirements needed for a specific community's health service.

It is clear that utilizing a patient care need "classification system," whether in acute care or community health, provides a more comprehensive mechanism for staffing and resultant fiscal management in effective use of nursing manpower.

REFERENCES

1. Stevens, B. J. *The Nurse As Executive* (Wakefield, Mass.: Contemporary Publishers, Inc. 1975) p. 132.
2. U.S. Department of Health, Education and Welfare, National Institutes of Health. *Nurse Staffing Methodology—A Review and Critique of Selected Literature* (Washington, D.C.: Government Printing Office 1973) p. 45–46.
3. *Ibid.*, p. 55.
4. Roberts, D. E. *The Staffing of Public Health and Outpatient Nursing Services—Methods of Study* (Geneva: World Health Organization 1963) p. 9.
5. *Ibid.*, p. 11.
6. *Ibid.*, p. 36.
7. Akin, K. "Work Measurement Studies in Small Health Departments." *Nursing Outlook* 10 (August 1962) p. 544.
8. Georgette, J. K. "Staffing by Patient Classification." *Nursing Clinics of North America* 5 (June 1970) p. 330.
9. Pardee, G. "Classifying Patients to Predice Staff Requirements." *American Journal of Nursing* 68 (March 1968) p. 517–520.
10. Price, J. "Patient Care Classification." *Nursing Outlook* 20 (July 1972) p. 445–448.
11. Tapia, J. A. "The Nursing Process in Family Health." *Nursing Outlook* 20 (April 1972) p. 267.
12. *Ibid.*
13. *Ibid.*, p. 268.
14. The Johns Hopkins School of Public Health and The Richmond Instructive Visiting Nurses Association. "Family Coping Index." (Richmond, Virginia, January 1964) Mimeographed.
15. *Ibid*, p.1.

Books for Nursing Administrators

Luther Christman, Ph.D., R.N.
Vice President for Nursing Affairs
Rush-Presbyterian–St. Luke's Medical
*   Center*
Dean of the College of Nursing
Rush University
Chicago, Illinois

Hierarchy in Organizations by A. S. Tannenbaum, B. Kavcic, M. Rosner, M. Vianello, and G. Weiser. San Francisco: Jossey-Bass, Inc., 1974. *248 pages. $13.95.*

This major study is concerned with the problem of power and its distribution in organized structures. This is what social organization is all about, and knowledge of the effect of social structure is vital to the construction of more effective organizations. The study of control and power has been the major research endeavor of the senior author, Arnold Tannenbaum. The other four authors are investigators from each of the other four countries—Yugoslavia, Israel, Italy, and Austria—that represent the other nations in this long-term, cross-cultural study.

The investigators studied large- and small-scale companies in each country, except in Israel, where only small-scale companies were included. The five industries chosen were plastics, non-ferrous founderies, food can-

178 neries, metal works, and furniture manufacturing. All companies were matched as closely as possible across countries though there were cultural differences in skill level, education, and sex ratio among workers and in hierarchical levels and span of control in organizational designs. Thus, the plan for matching plants had to undergo some compromise.

Some easily observed constants are found in all forms of organization. First, authority is distributed hierarchically; second, persons at upper levels are assigned more status and exercise more power and control than those at lower levels; third, having some "say" contributes to involvement; and fourth, persons at higher levels have more interesting and less repetitious jobs which permit greater individuality. The reverse of this condition exists at lower levels and is the cause of much frustration.

In the study, each member of the sample was examined for his distance from the top—the function of the number of persons intervening between him and the top. Each member had a second score which was the distance from the bottom. This varied from plant to plant due to differences in hierarchical arrangement because the chains differed in length.

Philosophical differences in worker control and participation differ with the cultures. In general, in the kibbutz system in Israel there is less stratification in hierarchical array and more participation by workers. All the workers were better educated and more uniform in technological knowledge than any of the comparative countries. The Yugoslavian factories were next in order of worker influence. In this country, dictatorship of the proletariat does not mean control by the workers but rather control on behalf of the workers. The United States falls into the median position. Influence of the workers is primarily focused on "bread and butter" issues. The Austrian hierarchical organizations are more to the right and permit less worker influence while in Italy the organizations are more patrimonial and workers have the least participation and influence. Thus, the kibbutz plants ranked first and the Italian plants ranked last on the survey questions on the decision-making items. The kibbutz plants are participative formally and informally. The Yugoslav organizations are participative formally and the American informally, while the Italian and Austrian organizations are participative neither formally nor informally with the Italian being the least participative on all counts. The Yugoslav and kibbutz plants have less dramatic, more "power-equalized" curves than do other plants, consistent with their more participative structures. The distribution of control in Italian plants is sharply hierarchical, as are the Austrian and American, although the Italian plants are not the most authoritarian because of the nature of ownership. Italian plants tend to be family owned and dominated. Management persons are usually selected from the extended family and thus movement up through the ranks is not generally possible.

The data revealed in this study have implications for traditional arguments about control and stratification in social systems. Some theorists have postulated that special rewards are needed to induce able persons to undertake training for crucial roles in systems and to assume the responsibilities of high rank. Nonetheless, kibbutz plants function effectively without a stratified system of monetary rewards. Furthermore, prestige seems to be of little importance. However, personal approval is highly valued. The investigators suggest that a normative model that advocates stratification of reward might therefore consider the problem of too much inequality as well as not enough.

Models of organizations cannot be divested from the larger social structure. They are colored by whether assumptions of common interest or conflict of interest prevail. The degree of participation may then become a self-fulfilling prophecy. The larger the scale of the organization and the greater the investment in costly technology, the more likely will the organization be set up to maximize the machines' contributions rather than to satisfy any ideological principle or a social norm.

The findings of this study suggest that social structure rather than interpersonal relations is the more substantial basis for understanding

outcomes such as the distribution of reactions and adjustments within a system. The cumulative effect of the mode of participation may be much more important than the personalities or the "human relations" management type of approach.

This study has much useful data for nurse administrators interested in organizational efficiency. The issues are presented clearly and it is worth the considerable time needed to ruminate on the findings.

Quality Assurance Programs and Controls in Nursing, by Doris J. Froebe and R. Joyce Bain. St. Louis, Mo.: C. V. Mosby Co., *1976. 161 pages. $6.25.*

The authors have done a commendable job in stating the main elements of a quality assurance program. The first part of the book, especially, contains clear, crisp definitions and illuminative diagrams. They seem to be at their best when examining the theoretical constructs of organizational theory that have lead to the present day state of the art. There is, however, one slight historical error re Max Weber. While it is true that one of his major works was not fully translated until 1947 he lived from 1864 to 1918. His theoretical work was well known in this country many years before that translation. The theoretical analyses, couched in historical sequence, should be very useful to nurses in orienting them to the reality of quality assessment—a fact of life

180   which nurses will have to recognize and deal with by imaginative use of scientific theory. It is interesting to note these author-administrators emphasize a strong clinical base as being a prime requisite for effective management and leadership in nursing.

The implementation section, the fourth and fifth chapters, is a "how to do it" section and is the longest portion of the book. This section contains a description of various protocols for the implementation of the quality assessment endeavor. A portion of this section is devoted to alternative strategies for staffing as an important principle in control of quality. In addition, a small section is devoted to means of facilitating communication.

The final chapter is allocated to speculation about the future. The authors use modern organization concepts and tie them into current developments in health care delivery to hazard their prognostication of alternatives open to nurses for more effective professional growth.

Medicine Under Capitalism, by Vincente Navarro. N.Y.: Prodist (a Division of Neale Watson Academic Publications) 1976. *230 pages. $14.95 cloth, $5.95 paperback.*

Navarro is an avowed Marxist and is a member of the faculty of Johns Hopkins University. In this volume he presents a Marxist view of health care. It should be made clear that his interpretation is very different from that prevailing in Russia and the so-called Iron Curtain countries.

Navarro asserts that the theoretical framework of Parsons and Rostow used in this country to explain underdevelopment of resources is incomplete. He asserts that (a) the cultural, technologic, and economic dependency of developing countries, and (b) economic and political control of resources by specific interests and social groups—the lumpenbourgeoisie and its foreign counterparts—are responsible for the general state of underdevelopment. He states that this phenomenon is equally observable in the underdevelopment of health care in large parts of rural America, as well as in foreign countries. Underdevelopment of health care is viewed as a direct corollary of the underdevelopment of all the resources of an area. He believes that underdevelopment is not conspiratorial but is a consequence of the internal logic of capitalism.

Navarro examines the flow of foreign-trained physicians as one of his postulates of the drain on capital resources of underdeveloped countries. His data show that the annual inflow of foreign physicians who entered the United States in 1970, 1971, and 1972 was far greater than our country produced in each one of those years. Of those who stayed and became permanent residents during the decade of 1960–70, 35 percent came from Latin America and represented an annual direct and indirect savings of $400 million. This is greater than the amount sent by the United States as annual aid for medical care and hospitals. That figure is estimated at $20 million. This decapitalization is particularly accentuated because there is a very high migration of physicians from some of the least developed countries such as the Dominican Republic.

Navarro devotes a chapter to the analysis of the underdevelopment of the health care of working Americans—he states it as the rediscovery of a forgotten majority. He uses coal miners and migrant farm workers as chief examples of poor occupational health provisions. His thesis is: The loss of autonomy is not in the sphere of consumption but in the production process itself.

He dismisses Ivan Illich's work as not having substance because he believes that a change in lifestyle is not sufficient in itself to bring about a better state of health and health care. He also concludes that the U.S.S.R. has problems similar to those of the United States. Referring to the former he asserts the central control imposed by the Communist Party to reinforce the power of the few is very similar to the way capitalism operates in this country. He believes neither country will achieve the kind of society that is desirable until democratization of resources occurs in both.

The section that may be of interest to nurses is the author's analysis of the health labor force. Navarro ties the data, not to the women's movement so much as the socioeconomics of men in the work force. He states also that a capitalistic society usually views women as a reserve work force to move in and out of employment as the economy demands. He quotes none other than Florence Nightingale as contributing to the definition of nursing as a support to the physician, mothering devotion to the patient, and a firm but kind discipline of attendants. He believes the television dramas support the stereotype of nurses as appendages to physicians. He extends his comparison of women being viewed in dependent jobs to the political-institutional arena because the decision-making bodies (boards of trustees) usually do not have much female representation. He notes, as an aside, that women physicians are more prone to support the status quo than to represent women in the lower economic groupings.

This book is worth reading to gain an awareness of how we might add to our perceptions of the strengths and weaknesses of our current system of health care.

Luther Christman, Ph.D., R.N.,
*   F.A.A.N.*
Vice President for Nursing Affairs
Rush-Presbyterian—St. Luke's Medical
*   Center*
Dean of the College of Nursing
Rush University
Chicago, Illinois

Path to Biculturalism, by Marlene Kramer and Claudia Schmalenberg. Wakefield, Mass.: Contemporary Publishing, 1977. *315 pages. $10.95.*

This book was written as a "map" for new graduates to use in straddling the cultural values developed as students with the values imposed by the reality of work. It appears to have more utility for baccalaureate graduates than for those who have finished other forms of RN preparation.

The authors have carefully summarized the main issues that confront nurses at this stage of their development. In a particularly well-organized sequence the strategy for making the transition from student to worker is related with keen insight. The authors, however, are quick to assert that professionalism requires lifelong learning. Part of the role induction into the work world requires the development of a growing edge.

The issue of interpersonal competence receives much attention. Scientific understanding and psycho-

184 motor skills are not sufficient by themselves. Nurses can be much more useful to patients and colleagues if they raise the level of human cooperation and are able to facilitate each other's work by keeping interpersonal tension to a minimum.

The book abounds with clever schemas that can serve as guides for nurses attempting to adjust to working immediately after being exposed to a different demand system from academia. The many line sketches vividly illuminate the concepts the authors are explaining.

The text should be of substantial help to students on their first job venture and to those responsible for orientation and in-service education.

The Geographic Distribution of Nurses and Public Policy, by Frank Sloan. Bethesda, Md.: DHEW Publication No. (HRA) 75–53, 1975. *214 pages.* $2.10.

This study was done by a small group of economists under the direction of Frank Sloan who, at the time of the study, was on the faculty of the University of Florida. This research study was designed to study the financial and nonfinancial incentives to improve the geographic distribution of nurses. The study includes: (1) a review of the literature on incentives that have shown to be effective in attracting nurses as well as other types of personnel to particular employers and a review of the experience of other government agencies in developing incentives; (2) an assessment of alternative measures of nurse distribu-

tion; and (3) original research on the geographic distribution of nursing services involving the collection and analysis of data from hospital directors of nursing and nurses on the staffs of the directors' hospitals.

The review of the literature on incentives is very complete and should be useful to nurses who deal with recruitment and retention of nursing staff. The basic factors covered are wages and income, fringe benefits, working conditions, characteristics that affect nurses' mobility and labor force status, job information and job search, and general environmental conditions. The review of the literature on nurse distribution complements literature on incentives and presents a fairly complete picture.

The chapters on turnover, nurse mobility patterns and attractiveness of various financial and nonfinancial employment centers cover a wide range of variables. Support data and statistical tables are supplied. The interpretations of the data are arranged in logical sequence. Nurses who read this material may have some of their opinions supported, but may have many refuted or have a new perspective brought into focus.

The final chapter contains the data on the investigation of nurse retention in current employment. In addition to the incentives usually studied, the characteristics of nurses and their families are included. The nurse characteristic variables prove to be more significant than the hospital variables.

A number of DHEW publications

are released with little publicity and fanfare that are very valuable to the field. This publication is in that category. The data compiled enables the reader to obtain a fairly complete understanding of the issues involved in nurse manpower. The information has a much more important use—informed persons should be better able to influence public policy more effectively.

Evaluation and the Exercise of Authority, by Sanford M. Dornbusch and W. Richard Scott. San Francisco: Jossey-Bass, Inc., 1975. *382 pages. $15.00.*

This volume is subtitled a theory of control applied to diverse organizations. The investigators studied a football team, a hospital, an electronics plant, a physics research group, a student newspaper, a university (faculty) and a Roman Catholic Archdiocese in trying to test the generality of their theory. The authors continuously made an effort to tie together theoretical developments and empirical studies. One of the values of this book is the alternation of a chapter on empirical studies with a chapter on a theoretical issue. The use of this interesting way of presenting theory and the real world endeavor makes for clarity of understanding and enables the reader to develop a growing sophistication with the difficult, and often hard to manage, field of evaluation.

The first chapter lays out the research strategy. The design is in the best tradition of research in complex organizations, straightforward and easily understood. The chapter on power is essentially a review of the literature in the field that the two sociologists used to formulate their theoretical approaches. They devote considerable space to clarifying their terms. They view goals as the desired state of an activity or set of activities. Goal setting in organizations is often accomplished through a continual bargaining process among shifting coalitions of the more powerful participants. Organizational goals are perceived as conceptions of desired end states determined by members in dominant coalitions. Goals are most likely to have consequences for the behavior of participants when they are assigned to specific persons. The discussion of task allocation and the accompanying activities of decision making, delegation, implementation, performance and outcome are excellent elaborations on these concepts.

A similar exposition of the concepts of tasks sanctions is included in this chapter. The entire chapter is valuable reading for nurses because of the insightful description of all the theoretical issues. The authors touch on an area of growing understanding among nurse managers when they state the "greater discretion permitted workers confronting active tasks must usually be coupled with greater individual competence, requiring longer training periods, if the discretion granted is to be effectively employed in guiding the selection and sequencing of task activities." When this condition exists, a smaller administrative

186 component can manage the planning, supervision and coordination. The empirical chapter that follows this theoretical discussion contains a number of examples taken from an analysis of nurses.

The chapter on evaluation gets at the nub of their theoretical concerns. They analyze the evaluation process with a clarity not usually given to this ambiguous activity. They take as one of their basic premises that performance evaluation is, by definition, an evaluation of a person. The factors affecting the evaluation process include task complexity, goal clarity and unpredictable tasks. The diagrammed model for the evaluation process is a helpful tool for grasping the theoretical notions. The empirical chapter includes a side by side analysis of the evaluation of school teachers and nurses. This comparative analysis is rich in information.

The chapter on authority in formal organizations is short but precise and contains two pictorial representations that summarize the content. Power is portrayed as one actor's attempt to control the performance of another by means of evaluations linked to sanctions. A fairly lengthy and elaborate discussion of the incompatibility and instability of authority systems is included as an accompanying chapter.

An authority system is perceived as being incompatible when a worker is prevented from maintaining an evaluation of performance acceptable to him. Incompatibility is a property of the system, not a characteristic of the worker. An authority system is unstable to the extent that it contains pressure for change. The final chapter is devoted to a theory of evaluation. All the previous data compiled in the volume are used to develop a theoretical framework that can be used to guide the development of evaluation strategy.

This book merits close study and several readings. It thoroughly covers a portion of the work world—evaluation—that is very troublesome for both managers and those who are evaluated. It contains many interesting concepts that could be included in an in-service program.

Employment Impacts of Health Policy Developments: A Special Report of the National Commission for Manpower Policy, Special Report No. 11. Washington, D.C.: Government Printing Office, 1976. *97 pages. Free.*

This monograph was written by Rashi Fein, in collaboration with Christine Bishop, and contains an introduction by Eli Ginzberg. The authors' interest is "in assessing past health employment trends, in questioning some traditional assumptions, in examining the directions in which health policy seems to be moving and in considering the potential impacts that these policies might have on the number and nature of the jobs that will be available in the broad area of health care in the future." They hope to set the basis for discussion among those responsible for manpower policy, those who formulate health policy and those who make fiscal decisions. The outcomes of the influence of these three groups have a profound influence because of the various ways the members of each group perceive the course of choice. Throughout the text the authors maintain a fundamental distinction between the two major types of health workers—those who are employed and those who are self-employed. The implications of a health manpower policy may have entirely different national patterns for both types.

The authors list four health characteristics: (1) psychological considerations, the feeling that the quantity and quality of medical care should depend on need and not personal income; (2) uncertainty, the unpredictability of the illness pattern; (3) individual's benefit from the next person's increase in health; and (4) medical care differences from other services in the consumer's relative inability to make quantitative and qualitative judgments of the services received.

The authors have a clear and well-organized chapter on the growth of employment in the health sector. The tables they utilize demonstrate the overrepresentation of women and minorities in the health sector. The vast increase in utilization occurred as a result of the combination of physician decision and third party presence. Increases in utilization were due to growth in the total amount of service and to increased complexity of care. Restraint began to be asserted when insurance companies found it difficult to raise premiums and government ran into tax dollar

shortages. Unions are starting to meet an impasse in bargaining for higher salaries because of these constraints. Prepaid group practice has the potential for reducing the demand for hospitalization to a considerable extent, and hence can cause possible unemployment of hospital personnel. If cost containment is pressed continuously, other alternatives for care may receive more attention. Home health care, rehabilitation, nutritional education and similar endeavors may be given more attention and thus change the type and quality of the work force.

From a purely economic analysis, this monograph has much to recommend it. That reasoning of the authors from which many nurses might depart is in the lack of tying the economics of care to the sociological issues of care. The authors observe repeatedly the employment opportunities for the disadvantaged, which they list as women and minorities. They have not differentiated clearly whether the care system has as its primary goal the delivery of health and illness care or whether the main goal is employment. If it is the latter, then two issues emerge immediately: (1) what are the quality implications for patients? and (2) must society face the same fait accompli about employment in the health sector as it now does in defense contracts?

The authors believe that managers will gain by cost containment policies. They assume that managers will have a stronger case for bringing in systems engineers and other experts. At the

188

same time they deplore the automatic ceiling placed on many of the task specialist types of workers and refer many times to the ladder concept as a desirable device. The inconsistency in their conclusions comes from failing to perceive that many of the task specialist types have emerged from the application of systems techniques, because attention was directed to narrow bands of activities that troubled managers, thus thwarting the flexibility the authors would like. Furthermore, on-the-job training is very much more expensive than generic training before employment. It is far cheaper to employ an all RN staff than to try to raise aides and LPNs to the level of RN competence through operational dollars.

Quality control is being mandated in several ways. The greater this pressure becomes the more likely will employers want skilled workers and the more the system will change to utilize trained persons. The issue of quality control may act as another barrier to the employment of the unskilled and semi-skilled. In addition, if patient complaints and malpractice suits can be lessened by employing the growing body of preservice trained persons, managers will be less prone to employ less than skilled workers. Unions may precipitate more turf problems instead of generating a

broader role for each worker. It will depend on what suits the economic outlook of union leaders than what is good for patient care. Instead of job enlargement it might be more useful to patient care to eliminate whole categories of task specialists.

The authors raise the caveat that with the growing attractiveness of employment in the health sector that white males may find employment in health care appealing and consequently be in greater competition with women and minority groups. This premise is not wholly false but it is only partially true. The authors fail to state that other forces may cause this attraction to occur. White males are facing either formal or nonformal quotas in the fields they once dominated. It may be out of desperation, not choice, that they turn to the health field. It is highly desirable that sex and race linkages to employment be eliminated but the goal will not be easily managed with scare words such as those raised in this discussion.

The authors conclude with a useful set of recommendations. They discuss the critical need to clarify national policy and give a better order of direction to a troubled sector of the economy. The information is useful to those who are engaged in designing new staffing patterns and new services.